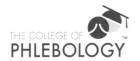

THE COLLEGE OF
PHLEBOLOGY

Advances in Phlebology and Venous Surgery Volume 1

Editors: Professor Mark S Whiteley, Emma B Dabbs

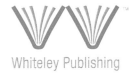

Whiteley Publishing

Published by Whiteley Publishing Ltd
First hardback edition 2017
ISBN 978-1-908586-04-9

Contents

Introduction

The last 30 years or so have seen a revolution in the understanding and treatment of venous conditions.

In the mid-1980s, the advent of colour flow duplex ultrasonography allowed healthcare professionals to visualise the flow of blood noninvasively. The ramifications of what this dynamic imaging technique has brought to venous surgery still continues. Not only did we discover that reflux is ascending rather than the previously assumed "domino" effect from above, but we also found that a good number (if not majority) of venous ulcers are due to superficial venous reflux and perforators and hence are potentially curable.

As the technology continues to improve, we are slowly getting to understand incompetent perforating veins and now pelvic venous reflux in the females, using transvaginal duplex ultrasonography. Unfortunately, due to anatomical considerations, the male pelvis and females unable or unwilling to undergo transvaginal studies still remain a diagnostic dilemma.

Just over a decade after venous duplex ultrasonography arrived, the advent of successful endovenous surgical techniques for the treatment of venous reflux gave another massive impetus to research and development in the venous world. Although endovenous surgery had been tried previously in different guises, it had never been successful enough to have taken over from traditional open surgery. The advent of radiofrequency ablation at the end of the 1990s, followed closely by endovenous laser ablation, completely revolutionised superficial venous surgery.

Since then, other endovenous thermal ablation techniques have been developed including steam, and more recently non-thermal endovenous ablation using cyanoacrylate glue or mechanochemical ablation have been developed.

The role of the pelvic veins both in terms of reflux for pelvic congestion syndrome, vulval and vaginal varicose veins as well as a source of reflux into leg varicose veins, as well as obstructive venous disease, has now become essential knowledge for anyone practising in the venous world. This book contains chapters on the diagnosis of pelvic reflux disease as well as pelvic obstructive disease.

This first volume of Advances in Phlebology and Venous Surgery contains a variety of chapters relating to the exciting changes that we have seen over the short history of endovenous surgery, hopefully exciting the reader into getting more involved into the subject of Phlebology. Each year, the COP College of Phlebology runs an international veins meeting in London in March, where like-minded healthcare professionals can meet to learn off each other, and to advance phlebology further.

Chapter 1

Endovenous thermal ablation of varicose veins and examination of the use and failings of linear endovenous energy density (LEED)

Author
Mark S Whiteley[1,2]

Institution(s)
(1) The Whiteley Clinic, Stirling House, Stirling Road, Guildford, Surrey GU2 7RF
(2) Faculty of Health and Biomedical Sciences, University of Surrey, Guildford, Surrey GU2 7XH

Introduction

At the most basic level, the treatment of varicose veins can be thought of as the abolition of venous reflux in the underlying venous trunk and the removal of any varicosities emanating from it (Figure 1). Of course varicose veins have become far more complex than the simple refluxing great saphenous vein or small saphenous vein with associated varices, with increased understanding of the role of the anterior accessory saphenous vein, incompetent perforating veins and pelvic vein reflux as well as the understanding of pumping mechanisms, stasis and outflow obstructions. However, for the majority of patients with uncomplicated primary varicose veins that present for treatment in vein practices, much can be learnt from understanding the most basic treatment of great saphenous vein reflux with associated varices.

In the past, following the original work from Trendelenburg at the end of the 19th century, doctors used to think that reflux emanated from the groin. The valves then failed progressively down the vein due to pressure effects from above, eventually causing dilation of surface veins and varicosities. This led to treatment by high saphenous tie. Of course, as we now know, this is inadequate and the introduction of stripping in addition to the high tie resulted in far better results than high tie alone[1]. The reason for this became apparent when it became clear that reflux is an ascending problem, not a descending problem[2].

It appears that reflux starts lower in the leg, with valves failing in a progressively upward manner. Not surprisingly, the high saphenous tie has now become redundant as it is clear that the ablation of reflux is the most important part of the operation. This is not only evidenced by the early work showing stripping to be superior to high ligation alone, but is also clear to anyone performing endovenous techniques. It is now common to start the ablation from the inferior epigastric vein,

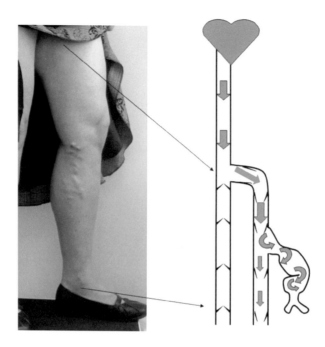

Figure 1: Left - Clinical picture and – right - stylised diagram illustrating truncal venous reflux, with associated dilated incompetent superficial varices (from: Understanding Venous Reflux: The Cause of Varicose Veins and Venous Leg Ulcers. Mark S Whiteley. ISBN: 978-1908586001).

thus completely avoiding anything resembling a high tie. Long-term success is achieved by successful ablation of reflux in the great saphenous vein trunk itself[5] (see chapter 4 in this book).

Despite the apparent success of stripping, the advent of endovenous thermal ablation questioned whether this is truly a gold standard for treating truncal saphenous reflux. Early in the history of endovenous thermoablation, doctors were attracted to the new technique because of the minimal access reducing the need for a wound in the groin with the associated pain and risk of potential infection, the reduced pain and bruising of endovenous ablation of the trunk compared to stripping of the vein and of course an earlier return to work and normal activity.

However, having started endovenous treatments in 1999, it became apparent to us by 2005 that the actual advantage was that the new endovenous techniques seem to result in reduced recurrence rates. This prompted us to look at the body's response to stripping of the great saphenous vein.

Fortunately, we had previously started a study trying to identify the role of the incompetent perforating vein and had started a randomised controlled study looking at patients presenting with varicose veins due to great saphenous vein reflux and at least one incompetent perforator. These patients were randomised to high saphenous tie and strip alone versus high saphenous tie and strip with subfascial endoscopic perforating vein surgery to incompetent perforators (SEPS). We had intended to show that the addition of the SEPS procedure, treating incompetent perforating veins, would lead to a reduction in recurrent varicose veins. However, any such effect that might be present was hidden by recurrence of reflux in the great saphenous vein tract.

As part of the protocol of the study, we had performed intraoperative ultrasound confirming the removal of the stripped great saphenous vein at the time of stripping, to make absolutely sure that there were no portions of retained great saphenous vein. Despite this, one year later we found that 23% of people had some element of reflux in the strip tract with 5% of people showing total recanalisation of the whole strip tract, which of course was incompetent and hence refluxing[4]. We won a local prize in 2005 for this work and published this in the British Journal of Surgery in 2007, suggesting that this strip tract revascularisation was perfectly explainable by previous work performed in wound healing from previous decades. Wound healing experts had long since shown that cut veins resulted in endothelial budding into the associated haematoma, solid cords of endothelial cells communicating with each other which then dilated into channels. These venous channels then coalesced forming veins. Of course no valves are formed in these new vessels.

In our sequential follow-up of these patients, we were able to show that in the strip tract, multiple small incompetent veins were formed as predicted by the research into wound healing previously. The British Journal of Surgery allowed us to publish this, but interestingly would not allow us to publish the histology that we obtained from one of these patients (Figure 2). This histological slide was reported as showing normal vein wall at a microscopic level, with the vein wall being surrounded by scar tissue. However, at a macroscopic level, the vein in question clearly showed four different lumens as shown in the ultrasound. Evidence that the vein grew back in its entirety rather than just being an endothelialized strip tract was too much for the referees to allow!

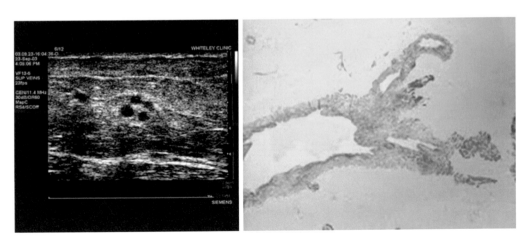

Figure 2: Left - B-Mode ultrasound image showing a transverse view of strip-tract revascularisation, evidenced by 4 lumens in the position where the previously stripped Great Saphenous Vein had been. Right - Histology of section of the same vein remove by surgical excision biopsy showing 4 lumens, histologically normal vein wall but vein surrounded by scar tissue.

Subsequently, we have shown that this process continues, and have published the 5 to 8 year results of this group which showed that 82% of patients had some evidence of strip tract revascularisation and reflux, with 13% having full strip-tract revascularisation[5].

Endovenous thermal ablation - mechanism of action and transmural death
Considering this data, we looked at our early results from endovenous thermal ablation using the early radiofrequency ablation device, VNUS Closure. Looking at our early results, we found no evidence at all of any neovascularisation in the groin nor any strip tract revascularisation[6,7]. Moreover, the treated great saphenous vein was virtually impossible to see at one year. Rather than showing any evidence of revascularisation, the thermally ablated vein showed atrophy.

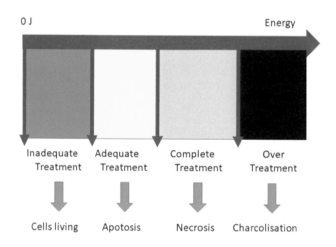

Figure 3: A diagram to illustrate the effect of increasing thermal energy from an endovenous thermal ablation device, on the cells in the vein wall. Apotosis and necrosis are the outcomes sought from endovenous thermal ablation.

Previously I had treated a section of stripped great saphenous vein with a radiofrequency catheter and sent the vein for histology. I published the results in 2004 in a chapter of a book, showing that the radiofrequency ablation had caused transmural death[8]. At that stage I first published my theory, repeated in a subsequent chapter for another book[9], that to cause permanent closure of an incompetent truncal vein with endovenous thermoablation, it would be necessary to kill all of the cells in the vein wall - i.e. "transmural death". Before this time, it had been thought that the primary mechanism of action of endovenous thermal ablation was protein contraction and any cellular damage was a secondary effect, and little attention was paid to whether the cells were alive or dead[10]. This is clearly incorrect as it is the death of the cells in the vein wall that causes long-term atrophy of the vein, the protein contraction only being useful to reduce the requirement for compression after treatment. If this were not the case, sclerotherapy would never work, as it kills the cells but doesn't cause protein contraction.

I suggested that inadequate treatment would result in damage to the inner layers only, causing thrombosis within the lumen of the vein. This, in conjunction with a "living vein skeleton" of media and adventitia in the outer walls of the vein would allow recanalisation in the medium to long term[8,9]. As I suggested at that time, this could result in failure of long-term "closure" after inadequate endovenous thermal ablation and also might account for recanalisation after sclerotherapy in thick-walled veins. This has been confused by some clinicians in the field who have mistaken "closure" by thrombus formation for permanent closure by transmural death and subsequent atrophy[11].

From this early work, we have developed an *in vitro* model for thermal ablation using porcine liver[12] and also have used *ex vivo* great saphenous vein to investigate the effect of different thermoablation devices on the vein wall[13]. What has become clear is that for transmural death, cells within the vein wall have to be damaged sufficiently to either undergo necrosis (due to protein degradation and instant cellular death) or apoptosis (where the cell itself or surrounding cells have been damaged sufficiently to stimulate the apoptotic pathway resulting in programmed cell death) (Figure 3).

Inadequate thermal injury to any of the cells will result in those cells surviving which may result in failure of atrophy and hence, failure of closure of the vein. Conversely, overtreatment of some of the vein wall will result in degradation of the cells and surrounding proteins, through coagulation and then necrosis of the cells and denaturation of the proteins, to carbonisation of the tissue. From an energy point of view, the extra energy used to cause carbonisation has been wasted as this energy should have been transmitted to cells further out in the vein wall.

Linear endovenous energy density (LEED)
Early practitioners in the field of endovenous thermal ablation soon realised that the temperature of the inner layer of the vein was nowhere near as important as making sure that the thermal energy

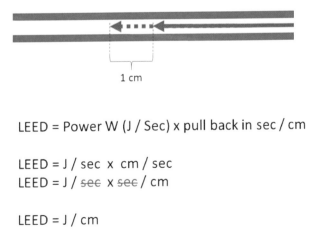

1 cm

LEED = Power W (J / Sec) x pull back in sec / cm

LEED = J / sec x cm / sec
LEED = J / ~~sec~~ x ~~sec~~ / cm

LEED = J / cm

Figure 4: An explanation of how LEED is calculated for endovenous thermal ablation (W = Watts; J = Joules).

required to treat the vein reached the adventitia[10]. It is surprising that the early VNUS Closure™ catheter had a thermocouple which rested on the endothelium as this could mislead surgeons into thinking an adequate temperature had been reached just because the inner wall of the vein had reached the target temperature of 85°C (subsequently revised to 90°C). Although these early clinicians were concentrating on adequate thermal energy to ensure protein contraction in the vein wall, it is fortunate that it is almost the same argument when considering adequate thermal energy to cause transmural death of the cells of the vein wall.

In 2004, Thomas Proebstle developed the idea of the Linear Endovenous Energy Density (LEED) to measure the amount of energy delivered to a unit length of vein by endovenous laser[14] (Figure 4). Although originally developed for the laser, this same measure can be used for radiofrequency ablation or indeed any endovenous thermoablation device.

As explained in figure 4, LEED is measured in joules per centimetre.

LEED is by necessity a fairly coarse measure, as it is only measuring how much energy is being transmitted from the device per centimetre of pullback. It is very useful during endovenous procedures because most devices allow the LEED to be monitored during the procedure. Provided the operator knows what power setting they are using, then they can modify the pullback rate to hit a target LEED for that section of vein.

Of course there are many criticisms of LEED. The first and most obvious is that it is assumed that all of the energy that is transmitted from the device is absorbed by the vein wall. If the operator uses good technique, this may be a fair assumption. However, if there is any blood within the vein lumen, some of the energy may be absorbed by the blood and is therefore not available to ablate the vein wall. It is also possible that using some wavelengths, energy may be lost by photons passing through the vein wall and not interacting with any chromophore within the vein wall itself, losing energy from the system and from thermal ablation of the vein.

Energy from endovenous device	=	**Energy absorbed by vein wall**	−	**Energy absorbed by any blood in vein lumen**	−	**Energy lost by failure to interact with vein wall**

Frequently when doctors fail to close veins at reasonably high LEEDs, it is due to them failing to exsanguinate the vein before treatment. This is frequently caused by doctors using a table that does not tip the patient head down, or if they do tip the patient head down then the angle is not severe enough. Furthermore, inadequate tumescence will also compound this problem. As the venous pressure in the leg is approximately 15 mmHg, a good general rule is that the patient is placed in a head down tilt before starting endovenous ablation, such that the saphenofemoral junction is 15 cm higher than the heart. Although in pressure terms 1 mmHg does not equal 1 cm of water precisely, it is a fairly good rule of thumb to ensure adequate tilting of the patient before treatment.

The second major problem is the volume of vein wall that needs to be treated. Although doctors

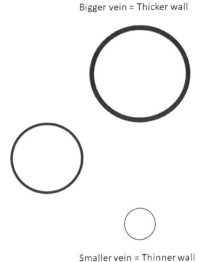

Bigger vein = Thicker wall

Smaller vein = Thinner wall

Figure 5: Diagram showing the usual relation of vein wall thickness and vein diameter in different veins. Generally, the larger the vein, the larger the vein diameter and the thicker the vein wall. Conversely, the smaller the vein, the smaller diameter and the thinner the vein wall. The volume of tissue in the vein wall is related to the circumference of the vein and the thickness of the vein wall.

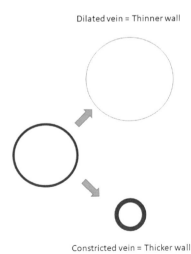

Dilated vein = Thinner wall

Constricted vein = Thicker wall

Figure 6: Diagram showing the usual relation of vein wall thickness and vein diameter in a single vein when it is dilated and constricted. When the vein is dilated it has a larger diameter and thinner wall; when constricted, the vein diameter is smaller and the veins wall is thicker.

get hung up about the diameter of the vein, this is actually irrelevant unless the thickness of the vein wall is also taken into consideration (Figure 5 and 6). The reason that doctors like to talk about the diameter of the vein is because this is easily measured on ultrasound. However, veins can constrict and dilate, changing this measurement. The target of the endovenous thermal ablation is the vein wall not the lumen. When considering how much energy is needed to cause transmural death, it is the mass of the vein wall that is important, not the size of the lumen.

This can be simply likened to cooking a chicken or turkey. The amount of energy required, measured in terms of temperature and time in an oven, depends on the mass of the flesh of the bird, not the size as the empty cavity inside the bird as this is irrelevant in the cooking process.

Hence, when doctors are producing protocols on how much energy they are using dependent upon the vein diameter, they are making an assumption that the vein wall is of uniform thickness which is actually incorrect. If one was to scientifically suggest a scale of treatment, then one should use the volume of the vein wall to be treated calculated from the diameter the vein and the thickness of the vein wall. This would then be a far more accurate measure of how much energy is required to treat the vein wall adequately.

Rate of energy distribution in vein wall - When reporting LEED alone is inadequate

Doctors and scientists working in the field of endovenous surgery quote LEED when discussing how much energy is required to close a vein. Indeed my own team has recently published a review of the optimal LEED required to obtain closure of great saphenous veins in different endovenous laser types[15]. However, even assuming that all of the energy emitted from a device is transmitted effectively to the target vein wall, is LEED the correct measure to report?

Figure 7 shows the problem. This graph plots power on the y-axis and pullback time on the x-axis. Each of the different lines on the graph represents one LEED. For instance, if you follow the line representing a LEED of 60 J per centimetre, you can find a multitude of different powers and pullback times that give you the same LEED. For instance, if you are able to find a laser or radiofrequency device that gave you a power of 60 W (i.e. 60 J per second) and you pulled the device back at one second per centimetre, your LEED would be 60.

Conversely if you set your laser or radiofrequency device to 1 W and you pulled it back at 60 seconds per centimetre, you would also get a LEED of 60.

However, anyone who has any experience whatsoever in endovenous thermal ablation will know that the effect of these two different extremes are completely different in reality, despite the same LEED. Also, both will fail to close the vein despite a LEED of 60 being recommended by many authorities.

The reason for this was shown in our paper looking at the effects of RFiTT in the porcine liver model and showing that if the energy level is set too high, then tissue adjacent to the thermal device is over treated, causing carbonisation. Scientifically what this means is that the rate of energy being passed into the tissue is too high, resulting in excessive absorption of energy in the near tissue and a failure of conduction of the thermal energy to more distant parts of the tissue. In a vein, this

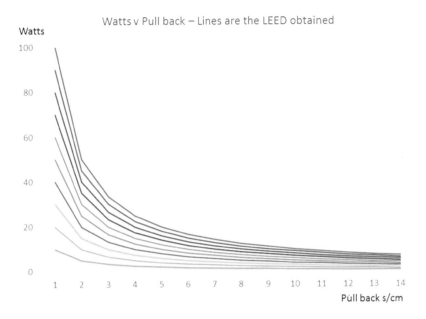

Figure 7: A graph showing the relationship between pull-back in seconds per centimetre (x-axis) and power in watts (y-axis) for different LEED's. Each line represents one value of LEED. The top line represents a LEED of 100 J/cm and the lowest line a LEED of 10 J/cm. The lines in between these two represent all of the intervening LEEDs in steps of 10 J/cm.

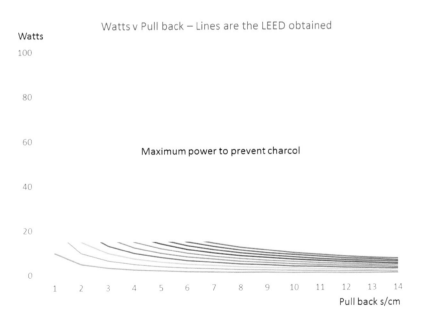

Figure 8: The same line graph as Figure 7, with suboptimal power levels removed.

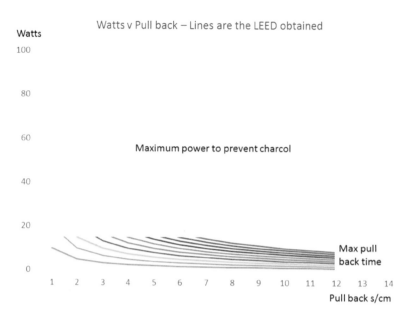

Figure 9: The same line graph as Figure 7 and 8, with suboptimal power levels, and impractical pull-back times removed

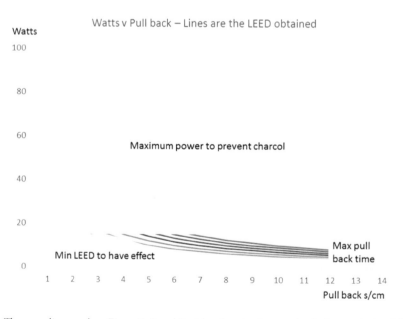

Figure 10: The same line graph as Figure 7, 8 and 9 with suboptimal power levels, impractical pull-back times and LEEDs that result in inadequate treatment are all removed.

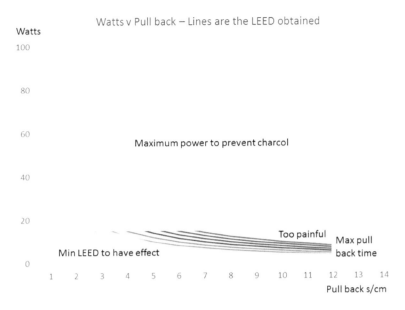

Watts v Pull back – Lines are the LEED obtained

Watts

Maximum power to prevent charcol

Too painful   Max pull
back time
Min LEED to have effect

Pull back s/cm

Figure 11: The same line graph as 7,8,9 and 10 with suboptimal power levels, impractical pull-back times, LEEDs that result in inadequate treatment and with LEEDs that cause too much post-operative pain are all removed.

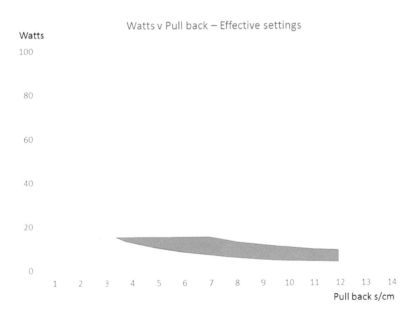

Watts v Pull back – Effective settings

Watts

Pull back s/cm

Figure 12: The range of combinations of power and pull-backs, which can be used for effective endovenous thermal ablation. As each LEED within this range can also be made up of combinations of power and pull-back that lie outside of this range, it is clear that quoting a LEED alone is inadequate. It is essential to quote a LEED with a power, or LEED with a pull-back to ensure that the LEED quoted is in the effective range of treatment.

means carbonisation of the intima with sticking of the device, whilst failing to ablate the media and adventitia. As such, we are able to remove suboptimal power levels from our target for adequate LEED (Figure 8). Experiments are needed to identify this power for each device, but generally 10-15 W is usually the uppermost level for an endovenous device where the energy emerges from a tip rather than having a long segment that is heated.

The next thing to consider is the length of time one wants to spend treating the vein. A pullback of over 12 seconds per centimetre starts becoming impractical (Figure 9). In addition to this, it may be that very low powers fail to have any ablative effect at all on the cells or proteins, as the heat may dissipate before any damage is caused.

From clinical studies, we know that low LEEDs, and certainly any LEED under a level of approximately 30-40 J per cm are inadequate to treat a truncal vein (Figure 10), and that high LEEDs especially over a 100 - 120 J per cm can be very painful (Figure 11).

When these limits are inserted into the graph of LEEDs, it can be seen that only certain proportions of each LEED line are included in what would be regarded as the effective range of LEEDs to ablate a truncal vein (Figure 12).

Therefore, to ensure that an appropriate energy has been applied to a vein by an endovenous thermal device, over an appropriate time period, it is clearly necessary to report the LEED and power together or alternatively the LEED and pullback time. Quoting LEED alone is clearly inadequate and is not useful scientifically.

Conclusions

Endovenous thermal ablation has become a mainstay of treatment for incompetent truncal veins and indeed since 2013, has been the recommended treatment for varicose veins by the National Institute of Health and Care Excellence (NICE) in the UK[16]. The major advantage of endovenous thermal ablation over stripping of the truncal vein appears to be the prevention of recurrence due to strip tract revascularisation, provided adequate ablation has been obtained.

Adequate endovenous thermal ablation requires transmural death of the cells in the vein wall, ensuring atrophy of the vein in the long term and prevention of recanalisation of any thrombus. Protein contraction of the vein wall is helpful as it reduces the requirement for any compression, but is not the primary reason as to why the veins atrophy.

It must be remembered that it is the mass of the vein wall and not the diameter of the vein alone that determines how much thermal energy is required for ablation. Hence, knowledge of the diameter of the vein alone is inadequate if the thickness of the wall is not also known.

The application of endovenous energy to the vein wall requires adequate energy at a rate that allows thermal spread throughout the vein wall sufficient enough to cause necrosis or apoptosis of all cells within the vein wall. Energy supplied too quickly (i.e.: at too high a power) can result in carbonisation of the tissue adjacent to the endovenous thermal ablation device, resulting in sticking of the device and inadequate treatment of the media and adventitia with an increased potential of recurrence due to recannalisation.

LEED is a useful measure of endovenous thermal ablation but is only useful if quoted along with the power or the pullback time used.

References

1. Dwerryhouse S, Davies B, Harradine K, Earnshaw JJ. Stripping the long saphenous vein reduces the rate of reoperation for recurrent varicose veins: five-year results of a randomized trial. J Vasc Surg. 1999; 29(4): 589-92.

2. Fassiadis N, Holdstock JM, Whiteley MS. The saphenofemoral valve: Gate keeper turned into rear guard. Phlebology. 2002;17: 29-31.

3. Taylor D, Whiteley AM, Holdstock JM, Price BA, Whiteley MS. Long term results of thermoablation of the Great Saphenous Vein – outcomes ten years after treatment. Advances in phlebology and venous surgery: volume 1. Whiteley Publishing Ltd. 2017.

4. Munasinghe A, Smith C, Kianifard B, Price BA, Holdstock JM, Whiteley MS. Strip-track revascularisation after stripping of the great saphenous vein. Br J Surg. 2007; 94 (7): 840-3.

5. Ostler AE, Holdstock JM, Harrison CC, Price BA, Whiteley MS. Strip-tract revascularization as a source of recurrent venous reflux following high saphenous tie and stripping: results at 5–8 years after surgery. Phlebology. 2015; 30 (8): 569-72.

6. Kianifard B, Holdstock JM, Whiteley MS. Radiofrequency ablation (VNUS closure) does not cause neo-vascularisation at the groin at one year: results of a case controlled study. Surgeon. 2006; 4 (2): 71-4.

7. Fassiadis N, Kianifard B, Holdstock JM, Whiteley MS. Ultrasound changes at the saphenofemoral junction and in the long saphenous vein during the first year of VNUS Closure. Int Angiol. 2002; 21 (3): 272-4.

8. Percutaneous radiofrequency ablations of Varicose Veins (VNUS Closure) Mark S Whiteley, Judy Holdstock. In: Roger M Greenhalgh ed, Vascular and Endovascular Challenges . London; BibaPublishing. 2004. p 361- 381

9. New Methods of Vein Ablation. Mark Whiteley. In: Venous Disease Simplified Eds: Alun H Davies, Tim Lees & Ian F Lane. UK: Harley 2006

10. Zikorus AW, Mirizzi MS: Evaluation of set point temperature and pullback speed on vein adventitial temperature during endovenous radiofrequency energy delivery in an *in-vitro* model. Vasc Endovasc Surg. 38:167-174, 2004

11. Lane TRA, Shepherd AC, Davies AH, 2012, It matters not a jot or tittle which method is used to thrombose the superficial varicose vein by heat - the result is the same, Vascular and Endovascular Controversies Update, Editors: Greenhalgh, London, Publisher: BIBA Medical, Pages: 546-552

12. Badham GE, Strong SM, Whiteley MS. An *in vivo* study to optimise treatment of varicose veins with radiofrequency induced thermotherapy. Phlebology. 2015; 30(1): 17-23.

13. Badham GE, Dos Santos SJ, Whiteley MS. Radiofrequency-induced thermotherapy (RFiTT) in a porcine liver model and *ex vivo* great saphenous vein. Minim Invasive Ther

Allied Technol. 2017; 2: 1-7.

14. Proebstle TM, Krummenauer F, Gul D, et al. Nonocclusion and early reopening of the great saphenous vein after endovenous laser treatment is fluence dependent. Dermatol Surg. 2004; 30: 174–178.

15. Cowpland CA, Cleese AL, Whiteley MS. Factors affecting optimal linear energy density for endovenous laser ablation in incompetent lower limb truncal veins – a review of the clinical evidence. Phlebology. 2017; 32(5): 299-306

16. NICE (National Institute for Health and Care Excellence) clinical guidelines - CG 168. Varicose veins in the legs: the diagnosis and management of varicose veins. Issued July 2013.

Chapter 2

Radiofrequency thermal ablation of varicose veins

Author(s)
Katherine J Williams
Ian J Franklin

Institution(s)
Academic Section of Vascular Surgery, Imperial College London and Imperial Healthcare NHS Trust.

Introduction
Venous radiofrequency thermal ablation refers to a technique developed at the turn of the century as a minimally invasive technique for the treatment of varicose veins.

Surgery for varicose veins
Varicose veins have traditionally been treated by methods targeting the saphenofemoral junction – a venous junction in the groin, where a very important valve, when working, allows blood pumped back towards the heart from the legs not to drop backwards under the force of gravity. Damage to the valvular structures of this and other valves in the great and small saphenous veins causes dysfunction of this ratcheting system, which can result in tortuous and unsightly superficial blood vessels in the leg, termed varicose veins.

Traditionally, the treatment of varicose veins was an operation called a saphenectomy, or "high ligation with saphenous stripping", where a cut in the groin was made in order that a surgeon may surgically disconnect the faulty junction in question. The rest of the vein down into the leg would then be destroyed either through hooking it out through many small skin incisions, or via saphenectomy. This operation can cause a lot of pain and bleeding, carries a significant risk of nerve damage in the leg and has a recurrence rate of 20-40% at 5 years[1].

Diathermy
In 1891, an American engineer called Nikola Tesla, first noted that irradiation of tissue with high frequency alternating current, at a frequency a little higher than that of radiowaves (i.e. radiofrequency ablation), produced heat[2]. In 1909, a German physician called Nagelschmidt coined the term diathermy, meaning "heating through", and suggested its potential for clinical use. He demonstrated

that electrical current with a frequency of greater than 10 kHz produced a thermic response upon application to human tissue. Since that time diathermy use has become widespread in many areas of surgery. Diathermy creates what is termed "electrocoagulation", which is where a damped sinus waveform of high-frequency alternating current is passed through biological tissue causing a heating effect. The movement of charge through resistive material produces heat at the area of highest current density. The current flows between two electrodes and the heat will be produced around the electrode with the smallest surface area. Hence, if the electrode within the blood vessel is very small surface area, whilst the surface electrode is large, the heat will be produced and dissipate within the vascular wall and surrounding tissues. Heat production is determined by current intensity and duration of application (Heat = current^2 x time) and decreases by the inverse square of the distance from the electrode tip (1/distance^2).

Vascular application

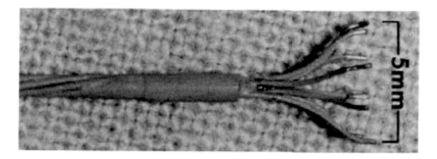

Figure 1: Endovenous diathermic vessel occlusion catheter. Taken from Cragg[4]

In 1972-82, Watts and Cragg explored the possibility of using a mono-polar diathermy-tipped lead, passed through the vein itself from a distant point and used it to create a blood clot to obliterate the passage of blood through the great saphenous vein in dogs and humans[3,4]. Termed endovascular diathermic vessel occlusion (EDVO), a catheter was constructed out of Teflon coated stainless steel with small bare tips at one end, flared outwards to achieve wall contact (Figure 1). The indifferent electrode was applied to the skin surface. A current was applied and the catheter tip pulled through a section of vein to be treated. In Cragg's study, venograms were used pre- and post-operatively and extravasation was seen in 2 out of 10 cases, one of which was a severe vascular tear due to catheter tip adhesion to the intimal surface and the other due to feeding the wire through the vessel wall. Recanalisation and collateralisation were prominent features in vessels two weeks post procedure and longer follow-up data was lacking. Watts described early intervention attempts in human subjects, combined with a high-tie and sclerotherapy, but at the time the procedure did not gain popularity outside the research arena[3]. Gradman advanced this to human clinical trials and, when paired with a saphenofemoral high-tie, termed it "venoscopic obliteration". He trialled it in 12 patients either by itself or with sclerotherapy and/or avulsions, with mixed results[5]. He declared a 33% success rate using the tie and catheter technique alone, whilst treating the rest with sclerotherapy and avulsions to achieve the desired effect.

Advances in the technique were slow to happen until 1998, when the concept of precise and delicately controlled heating (now termed "radiofrequency thermal ablation" or RFA), rather than total vein desiccation, was realised through the incorporation of a bipolar electrode with impedance feedback. Put simply, by measuring the resistance to the electrical current the output could be adjusted to deliver exactly the right amount of heat energy and feedback to warn if electrode wall contact was lost. Tumescent infusion of saline with local anaesthetic around the target vessel limited conduction of heat to neighbouring structures, most importantly to protect adjacent nerve and skin from thermal damage.

Two competing catheter device designs were developed by VNUS at this time – the Restore[TM] and the Closure[TM] devices. Both delivered heat energy specifically to the vein wall and vein contact temperature was precisely controlled via the placement of microthermocouples on the electrodes. Induction of heat in the venous intima causes collagen denaturation and contraction/luminal ablation.

- ### Restore[TM] catheter

Figure 2a

The catheter contained a central lumen for fluid infusion and the option of passage over a guide wire. There was a central un-insulated electrode with expansile longitudinal electrodes that expanded in a radial direction when in place, providing resistance to counter uncontrolled vein wall shrinkage (Figure 2). The catheter was placed within 1 cm of the base of a refluxing valve that had been proven on duplex scanning to be competent when compressed to a certain diameter ("the competence diameter"). This is the diameter at which the annulus of the mobile but non-occlusive leaflets narrowed restoring leaflet approximation and reflux was abolished. Once the catheter was in place blood flow was excluded from the treatment section by compression of groin tributaries and compression wrapping of the limb from the foot to groin. Electrodes were deployed and good wall contact was confirmed by impedance testing. Heating at 72°C and gradually collapsing the electrodes

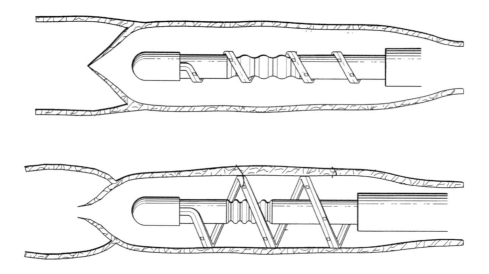

Figure 2b

Figure 2: two designs of Restore catheter (a+b). By heating the vein wall close to the valve annulus, contraction of collagen denaturation from bundle to coil shaped causes constriction of the vein calibre, allowing dilated valve leaflets to oppose and function again.
(b modified from www.freepatentsonline.com)

whilst maintaining wall contact caused limited constriction. The target diameter was predetermined as 1 mm less than the competence diameter. The restorative procedure avoided thrombus plug formation at the electrodes by treatment with peri- and post-operative heparin and post-treatment measures to augment deep venous flow, such as knee length support hose, supervised or programmed walking and avoidance of prolonged sitting and standing.

- **Closure™ catheter**

The concept behind the Closure™ catheter as opposed to the Restore™, was to cause contraction and ablation of the targeted vein section. In this way, blood was diverted through the deep veins through a competent valvular system. Again, the design incorporated collapsible bipolar electrodes, available in two diameter sizes which were exposed by pulling back a catheter sheath, around a hollow central catheter (Figure 3). Through this, heparinised saline could be infused to minimise clot formation on the catheter tip. Impedance feedback ensured even heating of the vessel wall to 85°C. Pre-operative ultrasound was used to mark the target vessel from groin to knee or ankle as needed and the vein was accessed either through a surgical incision or percutaneous venepuncture using the Seldinger technique. The catheter was introduced into the vein and peri-operative Doppler ultrasound confirmed correct catheter placement. The leg was elevated and exsanguinated – originally with a rubber Esmarch bandage and later by tumesence. Manual pressure was applied to the venous system at the groin and the diathermy power source activated. Slow drawback heating along the vein

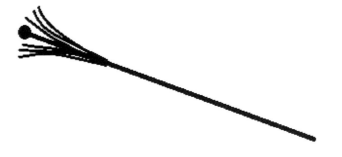

Figure 3a

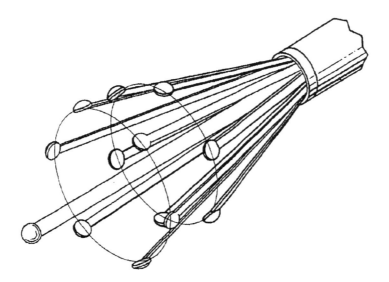

Figure 3b

Figure 3: Closure™ catheter design with expanding but compressible electrodes to aid wall contact for even heating. A sheath is withdrawn once catheter tip position is confirmed with ultrasound to expose the electrodes. Microcouple feedback ensures an even operating temperature of ~85°C is maintained.
(b modified from www.freepatentsonline.com)

segment at a rate of 2-3cm/min once an operating temperature of 85-90°C had been reached aimed to achieve complete luminal closure and scarring. When the catheter crossed an ostium or tributary the operating temperature dropped rapidly. At this point the catheter was slowed to allow thermal equilibrium to re-establish at the operating temperature. The treatment minimised wall relaxation by leaving behind a small thrombus plug in the contracted de-endothelialised lumen. Phlebectomies and/or sclerotherapy could also be undertaken at the time of procedure or at a later date. Gauze and compressive dressings maintained pressure on the treated vessel and aimed to assist obliteration and scar formation.

In 2000, Goldman's small trial of the Closure catheter in 10 patients and 12 limbs reported a return to normal activities of daily living within 24 hours for all patients, 8 developed transient skin purpura for 1-2 weeks and all had complete resolution with no recurrences at 3 and 6 months[6]. Chandler et al. performed a much larger study (301 limbs) partially combined with saphenofemoral high tie and/ or avulsions and achieved a 96% acute occlusion rate[7]. Complications included superficial phlebitis (6.6%), parasthaesia (15% confined to upper leg, 30% in below knee procedures), skin burns (2.7%) and deep vein thrombosis (1%). At a mean follow-up of 4.9 months there was a 92% reported success rate.

Both the Restore™ and the Closure™ catheters were trialled against each other by the Endovenous Management Study Group[8]. The Closure™ technique with heparinised saline infusion and continuous catheter pullback at 2.5 – 3 cm/min, was compared to Restore™ technique with pre- and post-procedural prophylactic dose low molecular weight heparin and peri-procedural unfractionated heparin infusion. Esmarch bandaging, for exsanguination of the limb during therapy, was applied in both cases. Closure™ treatment caused acute obliteration in 141 (93%) of 151 limbs and Restore™ treatment acutely reduced reflux to less than 1 second in 41 (60%) of 68 limbs. Closure™ treatments were associated with early recanalization (6%), parasthaesias (thigh 9%; leg 15%; p<0.001), 3 skin burns and 3 deep-vein thrombus extensions, with 1 pulmonary embolus. Restore™ treatments were thrombogenic (16%) despite prophylactic anticoagulation and treated valves enlarged over 6 weeks, becoming less competent. At 6 months follow-up 75% of Closure™ patients were symptom free and 96% of treated limbs were reflux free. However 45% of Restore™ patients were symptom free and only 19% of limbs had less than 1 second reflux. From this the group deemed that the Closure™ technique, with further technical modifications could be as comparatively effective as a saphenectomy, whereas Restore™ was ineffective and problematic given the clinical results.

The technique today

There are two "next generation" RFA catheters in general use, one which is pulled back segmentally (VNUS ClosureFAST™) and one which is pulled back continuously (Celon RFITT™).

The more popular in the UK is the VNUS ClosureFAST™ system (Figure 4). It consists of a catheter with a 7 cm long tip with an operating temperature of 120°C. The first 7cm of vein is treated with two heat cycles (twenty seconds each) and the catheter then repositioned to the adjacent segment guided by marks on the catheter sheath in 6.5cm increments, allowing a 5mm overlap of heated vein segments. Total treatment time is very quick, a couple of minutes is standard for the treatment of truncal veins and this is one of the major advantages of this technique. Less popular but in current use is the RadioFrequency Induced ThermoTherapy (Celon AG Medical Instruments, Germany) or RFITT™ Procurve catheter. Introduced to the European market in 2007, operation of the 5Fr catheter is via a continuous pull-back method of 0.7 - 1cm/sec. An audible impedance feed-back signal allows the operator to vary the speed of pull back according to the adequacy of energy delivered, but may result in less reproducible results when compared to segmental ablation. The catheter lacks a central guide wire channel, which may make negotiation of tortuous veins

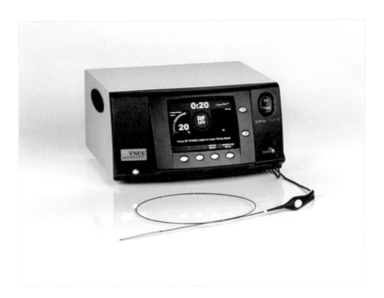

Figure 4 – VNUS ClosureFAST™ catheter with power source

difficult. RFITT™ has a slightly lower operating temperature when compared to ClosureFAST™ and when the operating foot pedal is deactivated endothermal ablation ceases immediately, much like endovenous laser ablation. The ClosureFAST™ catheter can take some time to cool down, which can become important if being used with local anaesthetic. An instant cessation in heating if anaesthesia is inadequate may reduce patient discomfort. At this point more anaesthetic can be infiltrated, or the catheter can be withdrawn slightly, before treatment is re-started.

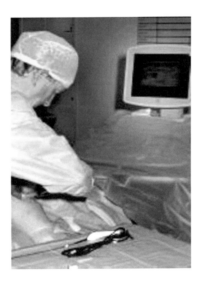

Figure 5a: Radiofrequency catheter, operating position and use of peri-operative ultrasound demonstrated. (Picture courtesy of Mr T Lane, Charing Cross Hospital)

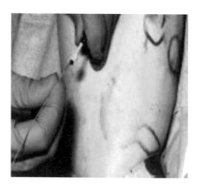

Figure 5b: Percutaneous insertion of catheter over a guide-wire (Seldinger technique). (Picture courtesy of Mr T Lane, Charing Cross Hospital)

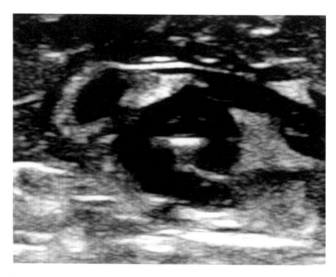

Figure 5c: Sonographic view of tumescence infusion, typical 'halo' appearance. (Picture courtesy of Mr T Lane, Charing Cross Hospital)

During RFA treatment external compression of the vein wall onto the catheter is understood to be important. This can be done with perivascular tumescence or compressive Esmarch bandaging. The use of a local anaesthetic and saline tumescence mixture minimises damage to surrounding tissue, ensures even heat dissipation and provides a short-period of post-operative analgesia. The ultrasound appearance of a tumescence "halo" can be seen in Figure 5. Post-operatively the leg is placed in compression bandaging to aid venous obliteration, reduce bruising and superficial phlebitis. This procedure is performed in an office or out-patient setting, with patients discharged home as soon as they are comfortable. Bandages are reduced after 48 hours to compression hosiery.

A 5 year European multicentre follow-up study looking at the long term results of radiofrequency segmental thermal ablation of incompetent great saphenous vein is due to report in the next few

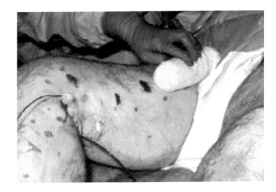

Figure 5d: Groin pressure applied after exsanguination of limb with catheter in situ.
(Picture courtesy of Mr T Lane, Charing Cross Hospital)

years. Preliminary results at three years show a 36 month occlusion rate of 92.6% and the probability of no reflux was 95.7%[9]. An improvement in clinical score (CEAP) was seen in 74.1%.

A seminal controlled randomised trial in 2011 by Rasmussen looked at 580 limbs (500 consecutive patients) with reflux of the great saphenous vein and randomised them to endovenous laser ablation, radiofrequency ablation, ultrasound-guided foam sclerotherapy and surgical saphenectomy under local anaesthetic and light sedation[10]. Patients undergoing RFA had no major complications compared to the other groups, where one pulmonary embolus occurred after foam sclerotherapy and one deep vein thrombosis after surgical stripping. Failure rates were similar for all modalities, but laser and RFA were associated with a faster recovery and less post-operative pain. Siribumrungwong et al reported statistically significant improvements in both clinical and health related measures of quality of life in their series of 200 limbs (148 patients), compared to surgery[11]. In multiple systematic reviews and meta-analyses, RFA has been shown to be at least as effective in the treatment of great saphenous varicose veins as high ligation and saphenous stripping[12,13]. These showed a lower risk of haematoma, wound infection and lower levels of perioperative pain compared to surgery. It also had statistically lower rates of neovascularisation and technical failure, with similar recurrence and recanalisation.

Radiofrequency ablation is a well-accepted, widely practiced method of treating superficial venous incompetence, and has been shown to be safe, cost effective and acceptable to patients. We await the long term results of the European ClosureFAST™ Clinical Study Group[9] with interest.

References
1. Stonebridge, P. A., Chalmers, N., Beggs, I., Bradbury, A. W. & Ruckley, C. V. Recurrent varicose veins: a varicographic analysis leading to a new practical classification. Br J Surg. 1995; 82, 60-62 .
2. In Encyclopaedia Britannica Online (2013).
3. Watts, G. T. Endovenous diathermy destruction of internal saphenous. Br Med J. 1972; 4: 53.

4.   Cragg, A. H., Galliani, C. A., Rysavy, J. A., Castaneda-Zuniga, W. R. & Amplatz, K. Endovascular diathermic vessel occlusion. Radiology. 1982; 144: 303-308.

5.   WS, G. Venoscopic obliteration of variceal tributaries using monopolar electrocautery. J Dermatol Surg Oncol. 1994; 20: 482-485.

6.   Goldman, M. P. Closure of the greater saphenous vein with endoluminal radiofrequency thermal heating of the vein wall in combination with ambulatory phlebectomy: preliminary 6-month follow-up. Dermatol Surg. 2000; 26: 452-456.

7.   Chandler, J. G. et al. Treatment of primary venous insufficiency by endovenous saphenous vein obliteration. Vascular and Endovascular Surgery. 2000; 34: 201-214. doi:Doi 10.1177/153857440003400303.

8.   Manfrini, S. et al. Endovenous management of saphenous vein reflux. Endovenous Reflux Management Study Group. J Vasc Surg. 2000; 32, 330-342.

9.   Proebstle, T. M. et al. Three-year European follow-up of endovenous radiofrequency-powered segmental thermal ablation of the great saphenous vein with or without treatment of calf varicosities. J Vasc Sur. 2011; 54: 146-152. doi:10.1016/j.jvs.2010.12.051.

10.   Rasmussen, L. H. et al. Randomized clinical trial comparing endovenous laser ablation, radiofrequency ablation, foam sclerotherapy and surgical stripping for great saphenous varicose veins. Br J Surg. 2011; 98: 1079-1087, doi:10.1002/bjs.7555.

11.   Choi, J. H., Park, H. C. & Joh, J. H. The occlusion rate and patterns of saphenous vein after radiofrequency ablation. Journal of the Korean Surgical Society. 2013; 84: 107-113. doi:10.4174/jkss.2013.84.2.107.

12.   Nesbitt, C. et al. Endovenous ablation (radiofrequency and laser) and foam sclerotherapy versus conventional surgery for great saphenous vein varices. Cochrane Database Syst Rev. 2011. doi:10.1002/14651858.CD005624.pub2.

13.   Siribumrungwong, B., Noorit, P., Wilasrusmee, C., Attia, J. & Thakkinstian, A. A systematic review and meta-analysis of randomised controlled trials comparing endovenous ablation and surgical intervention in patients with varicose vein. Eur J Vasc Endovasc Surg. 2012; 44: 214-223, doi:10.1016/j.ejvs.2012.05.017.

Chapter 3

Treating veins with monopolar radiofrequency – experience and results of the EVRF system

Author
Attila Szabó

Institution
Semmelweis University Budapest, Hungary

Introduction

Radiofrequency ablation (RFA) is a medical procedure, where part of the electrical conduction system of the heart, tumor or other dysfunctional tissue is ablated using the heat generated from the high frequency alternating current. RFA has become increasingly accepted in the last 15 years with promising results.[1]

Endovenous ablation has replaced stripping and ligation as the technique for elimination of saphenous vein reflux. One of the endovenous techniques is a radiofrequency based procedure. Newer methods of delivery of radiofrequency were introduced in 2007. Endovenous procedures are far less invasive than surgery and have lower complication rates. The procedure is well tolerated by the patients, and it produces good cosmetic results. Excellent clinical results are seen at 4-5 years, and the long-term efficacy of the procedure in now known with 10 years of experience.[2,3]

The radiofrequency ablation of varicose veins is based on thermocoagulation. The principle of thermocoagulation is heating the vein which makes it coagulate. This rise in temperature to 70-100 degrees Celsius is achieved by sending a high frequency pulse into the tip of the catheter or needle. Because of the rise in temperature the proteins in the vessel wall will solidify and make the vein disappear. Due to the isolation of the catheters the effect is very local, causing minimal damage to the surrounding tissue.

Immediately after endothermal vein treatment, biopsy specimens show a significant reduction in the size of the vein lumen, with denudation of endothelium, thrombus formation, thickened vessel walls, loss of collagen birefringence, and inflammatory changes. The zone of thermal damage is limited to 2 mm beyond the point of contact with the electrodes. Picture 1 shows the histology of the vein lumen one hour after endovenous ablation: the acute loss of endothelium is apparent. On Picture 2, 6 weeks after the endothermal procedure thrombus formation in the vein lumen and fibroblast migration to the intramural thrombosus is clearly visable.[4]

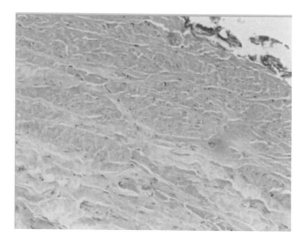

Picture 1: One hour after endovenous ablation (Source: Ronald Bush: Effects of Ablation on the Venous Wall, 4th Venous Symposium, NYC 2012)[4]

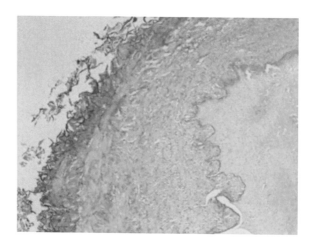

Picture 2: Histology at 6 weeks after endovenous ablation (Source: Ronald Bush: Effects of Ablation on the Venous Wall, 4th Venous Symposium, NYC 2012)[4]

The EVRF monopolar radiofrequency thermocoagulation system

The Belgian F care systems introduced EVRF (TC3000, in other countries VeinWave, now called ThermaVein) (see Picture 3) for trans-dermal treatments 15 years ago. It worked on 4 MHz and used 6-12 Watts, depending on the localisation and size of the treated vein. It provided an effective closure of small dermal veins with minimal heat transfer to the surrounding tissues, causing minimal damage, no pain and providing an excellent closure rate.

In 2009 F care systems developed an all-in-one device for the treatment of all sorts of varicose veins (Picture 4). With EVRF blue/red spider veins up to 1 mm, varicose veins from 2 to 5 mm (collateral, reticular and perforating veins), great and small saphenous veins (up to 20 mm diameter) and also hemorrhoids can be treated. The EVRF monopolar radiofrequency device produces a continuous output signal with a base frequency of 4 MHz, at maximum power it generates 25 Watts. This power is self-regulating and load-independent. At various loads – because physical characteristics of patients are different – the output signal shall be adjusted to reach the 25 Watts output. The measurement of the output signal is displayed on the screen in Joules per second. As previously mentioned, the output signal has a base frequency of 4 MHz, but the signal also contains a few higher harmonics for a more efficient feedback to the mass. That is why the patient cannot be grounded to the earth or

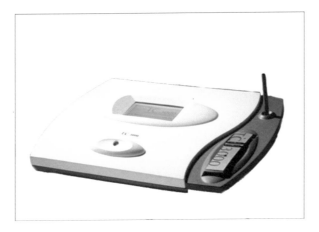

Picture 3: the TC3000 thermocoagulation device from F Care Systems

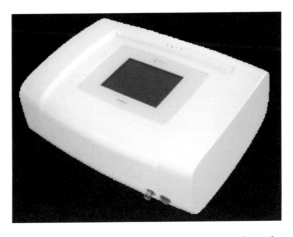

Picture 4: EndoVenous RadioFrequency (EVRF) 3 in 1 thermocoagulation device from F Care Systems

connected to other radiofrequency devices.

Small veins (up to 1 mm) on the face or on the legs are treated transcutaneously with a needle holder in combination with the special designed thermocoagulation needles:

- K3i needle with diameter 0.075mm (mostly used for facial treatment)
- K6i needle with diameter 0.150mm (mostly used for treatment of legs)

With the extremely sharp needle tip, the treatment is almost painless and causes only very light stains that completely disappear within a few days. The treatment causes very little to no bruising or swelling (Picture 5).

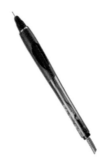

Picture 5: Handpiece for the treatment of reticular veins, teleangiectasias, capillaries and rosacea with K3i and K6i needles with TC3000 or EVRF

Varicose veins, tributaries from 1 to 5mm are treated with a specially designed hand catheter. The catheter is manipulated with a sterilized handset. Scrolling the handset's wheel will move the catheter into or out of the vein (Picture 6). These handsets are easy to hold and control, very flexible and the insulation makes it possible to slide the catheter into a varicose vein and coagulate the vein from inside. The catheter will be inserted into the vein and retracted step by step until the vein is completely closed. This thermocoagulation effect is similar to the treatment of the Great Saphenous Vein (GSV).

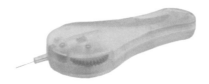

Picture 6: Hand catheter for the treatment of small varicose veins (1 to 5 mm) with EVRF

For the treatment of the GSV, the CR45i catheter is used. Its 5mm non-isolated tip and its flexibility allow for a smooth insertion. The catheter is pulled back gradually until the entire vein is closed. This procedure will take about 5 minutes. The treatment is minimally invasive, preventing unpleasant and possibly unsafe side effects such as pigmentation defects, superficial thrombophlebitis or deep venous thrombosis (DVT). Patients experience minimal discomfort and normal daily activities can usually be resumed within one day (Picture 7).

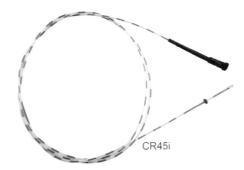

Picture 7: CR45i endovenous catheter for the treatment of vein trunks and large perforators with EVRF

Treatments of telangiectasias on the lower limb and on the face with K3i and K6i needles

Telangiectasias are permanent dilatations of small blood vessels near the surface of the skin or mucous membranes, measuring between 0.08 and 1 millimeter in diameter. They can develop anywhere on the body but are commonly seen on the face around the nose, cheeks, and chin. They can also develop on the legs, specifically on the upper thigh, below the knee joint, and around the ankles. Telangiectasias can be associated with varicose vein disease, but not necessarily. More than 50 % of the patients having telangiectasias do not have larger varices, and 15 % of the patients having advanced varicose vein disease do not have telangiectasias.

Sclerotherapy is the gold standard therapeutic approach for the treatment of reticular veins and telangiectasias over 0.3 mm. But for the ones smaller than 0.3 mm, there are other options such as thermocoagulation with radiofrequency and laser energy. With the selection of the proper laser type and wavelength lasers are most useful in the treatment of small red spider veins, but laser treatment may be more painful[5,6,7].

The thermocoagulation (radiofrequency energy) method is one of the alternative modalities that have been in use for more than 8 years, for the treatment of small reticular and telangiectasic varicosities that can not be treated by sclerotherapy. The main principle in the thermocoagulation method is a thermal damage that has been formed by a 4 MHz radiofrequency wave. When it is applied on a given lesion, it causes a 70°C temperature inside the treated vessel. As a result, plasma proteins are coagulated and parietal structures are destroyed. Thermocoagulation is a user-friendly, simple method and can be applied in large numbers according to the patient's and doctor's patience.

Small veins (up to 1 mm) on the face or on the legs are treated transcutaneously with a needle holder in combination with the specially designed thermocoagulation needles - the K3i needle with a diameter of 0.075 mm (mostly used for the treatment of facial veins) or the K6i needle with a diameter of 0.0150 (mostly used for treatment of leg veins). With the extremely sharp needle tip, the treatment is almost painless and causes only very light stains that completely disappear within a few days (Pictures 8-10). The treatment causes very little to no bruising or swelling. The needle is made of nickel. There are also golden needles available for patients with nickel allergy.

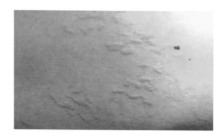

Picture 8: Oreols immediately after RF treatment

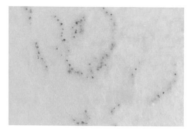

Picture 9: Crusts following RF treatment

Picture 10: Healed lesion

The selection of needle type is made according to the lesion, and it is attached to the handpiece. The energy level and the duration of impulses are adjusted. For face treatments 6-7 W and 0.2s pulses, for lower limb telangiectasias 9-11 W and 0.3-0.4s pulses are usually used. Patients are positioned supine or prone depending on the position of the treated lesion. No local cooling is used, because it could cause spasm and the smallest vessels would disappear from view. The tip of the needle touches the skin (but does not penetrate the skin!) and energy is delivered by pressing on the footswitch. There should be 1-2 mm distance between each pulse of energy. Lesser distance may cause the prolongation of the recovery time, while longer distance may decrease the success rate. There is no need for compression stockings or bandages after the treatment.

Treated lesions become flushed and swollen immediately after the RF therapy. These new lesions are called oreols (Picture 8). One day later these oreols vanish and are replaced by crusts (Picture 9). After a mean period of four weeks (1 to 8 weeks) these crusts peel spontaneously and completely resolve (Picture 10). In patients with skin phototype I and II, once the crusts have peeled off, a pale, white, slightly raised scar remains. These lesions lasted 1-3 months and then completely resolve.

Dr. Jean Marc Chardonneau in France reported the treatment of 5000 cases of small reticular and telangiectatic varicosities by TC3000 radiofrequency handpiece and K6i needles. In total he treated 19885 lesions in 5000 cases. The treated lesions were divided into 4 groups as Group 1: linear, Group 2: spider, Group 3: arborized and Group 4: papillary lesions. Recovery levels of each group were compared. Lesions were also classified according to their localization: anterior thigh, lateral thigh, medial knee, lateral knee, calf, ankle, foot. Patients were evaluated according to 5 recovery levels:

Level 0: <25% recovery,
Level 1: 25-50% recovery,
Level 2: 50-75% recovery,
Level 3: 75-90% recovery,
Level 4: 90-100 % recovery.

Result of the recovery levels of the four types of lesions after one treatment are detailed in Figure 1.

Lesions were also evaluated according to their locations. Recovery-levels of the lesions located below the knee, ankle and feet were better than the lesions located to over the knee especially lateral thigh. Recovery-levels according to the locations are summarized in Figure 2.

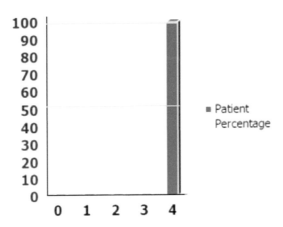

Figure 1a: Recovery level of linear lesions after 1 treatment

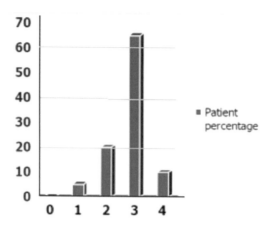

Figure 1b: Recovery levels of spider lesions after 1 treatment

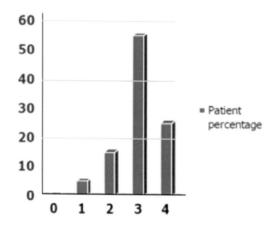

Figure 1c: Recovery levels of arborized lesions after 1 treatment

Between July 16, 2011 and April 20, 2013, at the Vascular Surgery Clinic, Semmelweis University Budapest, Hungary we performed 1500 treatment sessions for telangiectasias and spider veins (smaller than 1 mm) with K3i needles on the face (20 cases) and K6i needles on the lower limbs. 99% of the treated patients were females with a mean age of 32 years. We used RF treatment or, in some complicated cases (230 treatments), combined the treatment with liquid sclerotherapy (polidocanol 0,5% or 1% using a 30-33 G needle) - in those cases sclerotherapy was used for the treatment of larger veins and feeding veins, and the RF treatment used at the end of the treatment to clear up the remaining small veins. No anaesthetic cream or cooling was used, we created a stress-free environment for the patient and found this was sufficient for the procedure. On the face we used the K3i needles with 6-7 Watts and 2 pulses, on the legs the K6i needles with 9-11 Watts and 3 pulses. On the lower

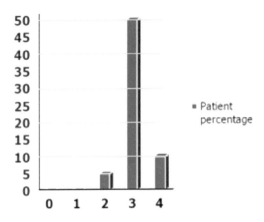

Figure 1d: Recovery levels of papillary lesions after 1 treatment

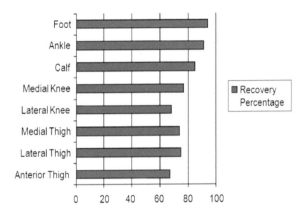

Figure 2: Recovery percentages after 1 treatment for lesions on the leg, according to their position

extremities a 0.3s interval was enough after some practice, while on the face we used 0.5s for more safety. The average treatment was 500 pulses per session, but in some cases we had longer sessions (2000 pulses). Recovery rate on the face was 100 % (3 patients - 15% needed a second treatment). On the lower limb we achieved an 82 % average recovery rate, 24 % needed several treatments. In the cases where sclerotherapy was combined with RF treatment, the recovery rate was 95 % after the first treatment session. The treatments were well tolerated, and we found that the pain level always depended on the patients' mood at the time of treatment. The crusts disappeared after 1-2 weeks following the treatments on average, however in some cases only after 2 months. 50 % of our patients felt an itching sensation in the treated area, which disappeared after 10-15 minutes. No side effects were reported. Patient satisfaction rate was high, and most of our patients come back for a check-up once a year.

The treatment of smaller veins (1 to 5 mm – reticular veins and small tributaries) with the CR12i and the CR30i catheters

The treatment of veins and tributaries (1 to 5 mm in diameter) is always a challenge for the surgeon. In many centers the treatment of the main trunks and tributaries is performed at the same time, while others treat them separately. Most of our patients request one treatment session. A wide range of methods are used for tributary treatments: microphlebectomy, sclerotherapy with foam, lasers of different wavelenghts and radiofrequency[9,10]. These procedures often have minor side effects: haematomas, bruising, pain, palpable thrombotic cords – all of these symptoms disappear completely over time, but they worsen the quality of life of the patient in the early post-operative period.

The CR12i and CR30i hand-catheters with EVRF are a perfect alternative for the treatment of tributaries and varicose veins from 1 to 5 mm (see Picture 6). The catheter is manipulated with a sterilized handset. Scrolling the handset's wheel will move the catheter into or out of the vein. These handsets are easy to hold and control, a very flexible and insulated catheter makes it possible to slide into the varicose vein and coagulate the vein from inside. The catheter is inserted into the vein through a cannula of the right size and retracted step by step until the vein is completely closed. The thermocoagulation effect is similar to the treatment of the GSV. For more superficial and deeper veins in the superficial compartment, tumescent anaesthesia combined with some compression is necessary to protect the surrounding tissue and to put pressure on the vein. The length of the catheter is 10 cm, thus for longer segments, treatment requires further cannulation points. The catheters are small and flexible, and easily pass through tortuous segments. EVRF CR12i and CR30i handsets provide a good alternative in the treatment of varicose veins ranging 1-5 mm in diameter.

Truncal vein treatment with the CR45i catheter

Management of varicose vein reflux has historically been treated with stripping of the GSV or Small Saphenous Vein (SSV), removal of the enlarged tributaries and interruption or ligation of the incompetent perforators. Since 1999, endovenous ablation procedures have been reported to be safe and effective methods for closing the enlarged and insufficient portions of the GSV and/or SSV, and even large tributaries, like the Anterior Accessory Saphenous Vein (AASV) and incompetent perforating veins (IPV). The endovenous methods provide faster recovery and better cosmetic outcome than stripping.

For the treatment of the GSV with EVRF we use the CR45i catheter. EVRF is a monopolar radiofrequency device, which works on 4 MHz and delivers 25 Watts of continous energy for endothermal saphenous ablation through the CR45i catheter. The radiofrequency catheter is 120 cm long, its insulation is made of PTFE. The 5mm non-isolated tip and its flexibility allow a smooth insertion. The catheter is pulled back gradually until the entire vein is closed. The EVRF device works safely when treating veins with a diameter of 3-18 mm.

The surgical procedure is identical to other endothermal ablation methods: in a sterile environment, the treated main saphenous trunk (GSV and/or SSV) or greater tributary (i.e. AASV) is punctured percutaneously with a 6 Fr sheath. The CR45i catheter is inserted and placed 2 cm below the sapheno-femoral junction (SFJ) or the sapheno-popliteal junction (SPJ)[11]. Tumescent solution (in our cases: isotonic bicarbonate 1000 ml, 300 mg lidocaine and 0.5 mg epinephrine) is administered under ultrasound guidance[12]. The characteristics of the catheter provide an excellent visibility under ultrasound even after administration of the tumescent solution[13] (Picture 11).

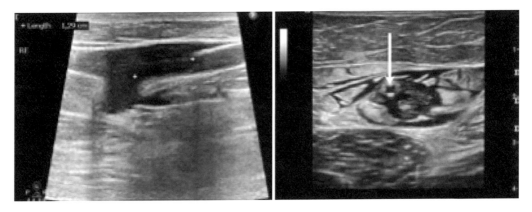

Picture 11: Left - EVRF catheter tip 2 cm from the junction[13]. Right - Catheter in the thigh region surrounded by tumescent solution[13].

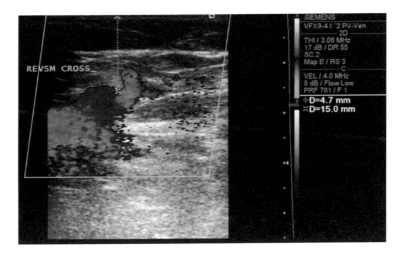

Picture 12: ultrasound picture on month after RF GSV ablation – GSV is closed

After double checking the catheter position at the junction, the RF ablation starts: 25 Watts continuous energy is administered, retracting the CR45i catheter every 6 sec/0,5cm according to an audible and visual signal. The energy used can be adjusted according to the vein diameter if needed. Generally 250-300 J/cm is used for the GSV. The RF energy targets the vein wall, it results in shrinking and collapsing the treated vein, creating a fibrotic seal and occluding the vessel. The treated vein is immediately closed after the procedure, its diameter reduces continuously over time and becomes a fibrotic cord in about 6-12 months. It is standard, in our practice, to apply a class 2 compression stocking after RFA, and patients can return to normal activity in 1-2 days. LMWH thrombosis prophylaxis is given for high risk patients. Clinical and ultrasound check-ups take place one week and one month following the RF procedure[13] (Picture 12).

Dr Sarah Thomis from UZ Leuven, Belgium completed the first clinical study on EVRF saphenous treatment with the CR45i catheter[13]. She included 40 patients with insufficient GSV from Nov 2011 to March 2012. Follow-ups took place at 1 week, 1 month and 6 months after the initial operation. The clinical data of the patients was as follows: mean age 50.1 years, gender 12/28 M/F, mean BMI: 25.2, commonest clinical reason to operate CEAP C2. The mean GSV diameter before the operation was 6.5 mm, the mean length: 37.2 cm. Total mean energy applied was 7365 J. The patients needed minimal amount of analgesia after surgery (mean number of doses = 0.7, mean days of oral analgesia: 0.9). Ecchymosis was measured and found to be very low. The mean duration of periphlebitis was 1.1 days, paraesthesia was found is 1/40 cases. Patient satisfaction was a mean of 8.9 (out of 10). The patient's quality of life showed a significant improvement after the EVRF procedure measuring with the CIVIQ-2 score, the pain score decreased from 2.5 at day 2, to 1.6 on day 7 and to 0.6 at day 10. The occlusion rate at 6 months was 92.5%. Dr Thomis concluded that the EVRF thermoablation procedure is safe and effective, and is comparable to other RF or laser ablation techniques.

At the Vascular Surgery Clinic of Semmelweis University Budapest, Hungary from July 16, 2011 to April 20, 2013 we treated 313 patients (99 men: mean age 47 years (range: 16-84 years) and 214 women: mean age 49 years (range: 26-79 years)) with saphenous reflux and varicosities arising from the GSV and/or SSV using the EVRF device with CR45I catheter manufactured by F care systems. The output power was 25 Watts, the catheter pullback speed was 6 sec/0.5cm with a double cycle at the beginning (12 sec/0.5cm), the tip was positioned 2 cm from the SFJ or SPJ. In each case we used tumescent local aneasthesia (modified solution: isotonic bicarbonate 1000 ml, 300 mg lidocaine and 0.5 mg epinephrine) with light sedation in the presence of an anesthesiologist, if needed. Depending on the patient's pain level we administered a low amount of midazolam, fentanyl and propofol to prevent pain caused by the injections used in administering the tumescent anaesthesia.

Patients' clinical data, the data of the pre- and postoperative ultrasound examinations, the total power emitted and the diameters and flow of the treated veins measured by ultrasound have been recorded. Photo documentation was taken in each case. Clinical evaluation was performed one day, one week, one to two months and one year after surgery using a scale of postoperative pain, VCSS clinical evaluation form, patient satisfaction and ultrasound evaluation of the veins treated during the procedure.[14]

RF ablation using the EVRF CR45i catheter from F care Systems was performed on 313 limbs - 268 GSV, 35 SSV, 10 GSV+SSV; 291 patients belonged to CEAP 2 or 3, 22 patients to CEAP 4 or

5; 274 primary cases, 39 recurrent varicosity. Crossectomy (ligation of the SFJ) was performed in 6 cases due to the GSV being larger than 20 mm at the junction. Tributaries were treated in the same session by microphlebectomy using a Varady phlebodissector and hook in most of the cases or using foam sclerotherapy with 1 or 2 % polidocanol. The mean diameter of the GSV was 6.2 mm (range: 4-16 mm) and of the SSV 4.8 mm (range: 4-10 mm), reflux more than 0.5 sec was detected with duplex scan in all cases. The length of the treated vein segment was 45 cm (range: 15 to 82 cm), using an average amount of 11320 Joules total energy. The average duration of surgery was 48 minutes, including the treatment of the enlarged tributaries by microphlebectomy[15].

Complete occlusion was found in 275 of the 276 cases (99%) at one month ultrasound control (until March 20, 2013), one GSV of an obese patient (160kg) remained open. At one year follow-up 3 of 108 patients showed recanalization longer than 5 cm (97.2% 1 year occlusion) without clinical

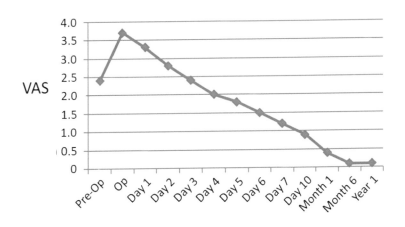

Figure 3: Postoperative Pain Score on VAS scale after EVRF treatment (own data)

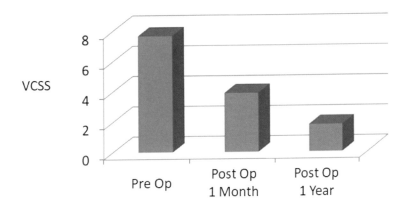

Figure 4: VCSS scores after EVRF treatment (own data)

symptoms. At one year follow-up we evaluated the postoperative pain reported by the patients on a visual analogue scale (2.4 preoperatively, 1.2, 0.4 and 0.1 1 week, 1 month and 1 year postop respectively), the VCSS score (7.7 before surgery, 3.9 and 1.8 one month and one year respectively) (Figures 3 and 4). The average patient satisfaction was 99% at 1 year. There were no cases of deep vein thrombosis, skin burns, neuritis or bleeding. We found minimal bruising at the treatment site of the tributaries in some cases, and 2 patients had mild inflammation, treatable with conventional anti-inflammatories.

Conclusion

New methods for the ablation of varicose veins have changed the concept of how we treat the disease. The advent of using modern ablation techniques has resulted in the classical crossectomy being performed less frequently, and classical stripping has been replaced by endovenous occlusion with thermal or chemical methods. The treatment of tributaries or smaller varices can be performed in one session together with the truncal ablation, though many surgeons still perform these seperately. All these new methods require a deep knowledge of venous duplex ultrasound. The venous duplex ultrasound scan is essential for the investigations and performing all the steps of modern procedures. Tumescent anaesthesia allows the operation to be ambulatory, so that it can even be performed safely in the surgeon's office.

The late results after endothermal ablation (laser or RF) or non-thermal ablation techniques (MOCA, Sapheon Glue) are comparable to coventional surgery, with signifcantly fewer side effects, less pain, much faster recovery and improvement of the quality of life[2].

With the help of laser or RF it is possible to treat telangiectasias smaller than 0.3 mm with success – these methods can easily be combined with liquid or foam sclerotherapy.

EVRF from F Care Systems Belgium can be used for the treatment of telangiectasias and reticular veins, using the handpiece and K3i or K6i needles (face or lower leg), small varicose veins or tributaries 2 to 5 mm with the hand catheters and for saphenous trunks and perforators 4 to 15 mm in diameter with the CR45i catheter. The only particular contraindications for the usage of EVRF are nickel allergy (golden tip needles available) and the having a pacemaker. In our practice the EVRF treatment with the CR45i catheter resulted in a 94 % one year occlusion rate, with no serious side effects and a high patient satisfaction. We found that the hand catheters were suitable for the treatment of smaller veins and tributaries. The handpiece with K3i and K6i needles proved to be useful in the treatment of telangiectasia, with excellent results. We found that the EVRF procedure is good in combination with liquid or foam sclerotherapy.

References

1.   Walker AE, Burton CV. Radiofrequency telethermocoagulation. JAMA. 1966;197(9):700-4.
2.   Rasmussen LH, Lawaetz M, Bjoern L, Vennits B, Blemings A, Eklof B. Randomized clinical trial comparing endovenous laser ablation, radiofrequency ablation, foam sclerotherapy and surgical stripping for great saphenous varicose veins. Br J Surg. 2011;98(8):1079-87.

3.	Health Quality Ontario. Endovascular radiofrequency ablation for varicose veins: an evidence-based analysis. Ont Health Technol Assess Ser. 2011;11(1):1-93. Epub 2011 Feb 1.

4.	Bush R. Effects of Ablation on the Venous Wall. 4th Venous Symposium, NYC 2012

5.	Tepavcevic B, Matic P, Radak D. Comparison of sclerotherapy, laser, and radiowave coagulation in treatment of lower extremity telangiectasias. J Cosmet Laser Ther. 2012;14(5):239-42.

6.	Schwartz L, Maxwell H. Sclerotherapy for lower limb telangiectasias. Cochrane Database Syst Rev. 2011;(12)

7.	Munia MA, Wolosker N, Munia CG, Chao WS, Puech-Leão P. Comparison of Laser Versus Sclerotherapy in the Treatment of Lower Extremity Telangiectases: A Prospective Study. Dermatol Surg. 2011 Dec 30. doi: 10.1111/j.1524-4725.2011.02226.x. [Epub ahead of print]

8.	Chardonneau JM: Efficacy and Results of Thermocoagulation Modality int he Treatment of Reticular and Teleangiectatic Veins: Midterm and Long Term Results of 5000 Cases.Available at: http://www.fcaresystems.com/clincal-evidence/clinical-trials/

9.	Harlander-Locke M, Jimenez JC, Lawrence PF, Derubertis BG, Rigberg DA, Gelabert HA. Endovenous ablation with concomitant phlebectomy is a safe and effective method of treatment for symptomatic patients with axial reflux and large incompetent tributaries. J Vasc Surg. 2013 Apr 6. pii: S0741-5214(13)00061-X. doi: 10.1016/j.jvs.2012.12.054. [Epub ahead of print]

10.	Kim HK, Kim HJ, Shim JH, Baek MJ, Sohn YS, Choi YH. Endovenous lasering versus ambulatory phlebectomy of varicose tributaries in conjunction with endovenous laser treatment of the great or small saphenous vein. Ann Vasc Surg. 2009;23(2):207-11.

11.	Feliciano BA, Dalsing MC. Varicose vein: current management. Adv Surg. 2011;45:45-62.

12.	Altin FH, Kutas B, Gunes T, Aydin S, Eygi B: A comparison of three tumescent delivery systems in endovenous laser ablation of the great saphenous vein. Vascular. 2013 Mar 19. [Epub ahead of print]

13.	Thomis S. Study on effectiveness of EVRF treatmentAvaiable at: http://www.fcaresystems.com/clincal-evidence/clinical-trials/

14.	Passman MA, McLafferty RB, Lentz MF, Nagre SB, Iafrati MD, Bohannon WT, Moore CM, Heller JA, Schneider JR, Lohr JM, Caprini JA: Validation of Venous Clinical Severity Score (VCSS) with other venous severity assessment tools from the American Venous Forum, National Venous Screening Program. J Vasc Surg. 2011 Dec;54(6 Suppl):2S-9S. doi: 10.1016/j.jvs.2011.05.117. Epub 2011 Oct 1.

15.	Harlander-Locke M, Jimenez JC, Lawrence PF, Derubertis BG, Rigberg DA, Gelabert HA: Endovenous ablation with concomitant phlebectomy is a safe and effective method of treatment for symptomatic patients with axial reflux and large incompetent tributaries. J Vasc Surg. 2013 Apr 6. pii: S0741-5214(13)00061-X. doi: 10.1016/j.jvs.2012.12.054. [Epub ahead of print]

Chapter 4

Long term results of thermoablation of the Great Saphenous Vein – outcomes ten years after treatment

Author(s)
Daniel Taylor[1]
Alice Whiteley[1,2]
Judy Holdstock[1]
Barrie Price[1]
Mark S Whiteley[1,2]

Institution(s)
(1) The Whiteley Clinic, Stirling House, Stirling Road, Guildford, Surrey GU2 7RF,
(2) Faculty of Health and Biomedical Sciences, University of Surrey, Guildford, Surrey GU2 7XH

History

Varicose veins have been medically recognized for thousands of years and endovenous treatment for them began at least as far back as 1682 with the injection of an acidic 'sclerotherapy'[1]. However, these early attempts at injectable sclerotherapy were largely ineffective. Surgical intervention with stripping and ligation of the saphenous system was first described by Madelung in 1884[2,3]. Invagination stripping using an extra luminal device was introduced in the early 1990s and went on to become the first truly beneficial treatment of varicose veins[4]. Tying off and stripping out of the incompetent Great Saphenous (GSV) and Small Saphenous veins (SSV) often provided a great deal of improvement in symptoms in the short term and so remained the mainstay of treatment for over a hundred years.

However, the procedure was invasive and led to significant trauma. It was also discovered that the severed ends of the stripped veins had a remarkable propensity to heal – with new (neovascular) growth of veins to replace those which had been removed. Neovascularization following traditional surgery has now been shown to be the predominant cause of recurrent varicose veins, which by ten years after treatment recur in up to 70% of legs[5-7]. The introduction of duplex ultrasound into the field of venous disease in the 1980s, later coupled with improved 'foam' sclerotherapy seemed to offer a potentially minimally invasive solution to the problems associated with stripping[8]. However, whilst foam sclerotherapy has been shown to be a highly effective mechanism for treating small vessels, it relies on direct contact with the vein wall, and therefore is less appropriate for the treatment of the larger truncal veins[9].

As far back as the 1930s, the delivery of heat was trialled as a means of treating varicose veins. However, it was not until 1998 when the VNUS Closure® device, coupled with duplex ultrasound, revolutionized venous treatment with the first successful introduction of radiofrequency thermoablation. This procedure was a minimally invasive, key-hole technique which delivered a catheter through a cannula under duplex ultrasound control into the lumen inside a vein. This catheter then delivered heat through the vessel wall from the inside in order to destroy it – with minimal trauma and no severing of the ends of the vein. After the VNUS catheter was inserted inside a vein it was pushed up to the desired position and then its flower-head arrangement of one forward and four lower electrodes (in the 5 and then 6-French Gauge iteration of the device) were opened up. Once this bi-polar arrangement of electrodes was resting against the inside of the vein wall, an alternating radiofrequency current was switched on. This current was conducted between the upper and lower electrodes via the vein wall and as it passed through, resistance led to excitation of the molecules and heat generation of approximately 85°C[10]. In order to maintain good contact between the electrodes and the vein wall throughout the procedure the patient's leg was wrapped in esmark bandaging for compression.

The heating of the vein wall led to the separation of the individual layers and the contraction of the collagen components of the intramural portion[10]. This resulted in the generation of fibrotic scar tissue and with correct application and heating temperature, histology showed that the VNUS Closure Technique resulted in complete transmural cell death of the treated vein[10,11]. As the VNUS catheter was pulled back continuously along the vein, the ablation of the vein wall led to its closure. The thermally ablated tissue of the vein wall was then no longer recognized as "self" by the immune system and so was destroyed by it over time. This destruction of the treated vein by the body was not only far less traumatic than surgical stripping – where smaller vessels connected to the target one were often torn out as well – but also resulted in a clean end to the treated part of the vein with no regrowth through neovascularization[12,13]. This lack of neovascular tissue following VNUS Closure eventually became the main benefit of the treatment over stripping, eclipsing the reduced trauma and near elimination of incomplete treatment that the technique, with intra-operative ultrasound guidance, also offered.

Thermoablation beyond 10 years

The keyhole nature of catheter based thermoablation, combined with the accuracy allowed with ultrasound, and the elimination of vein transection and subsequent neovascularization led to excellent short term results for VNUS Closure[12-15]. However, after over a hundred years of vein stripping there was widespread resistance to the new procedure. Many felt that burning a vein in order to close it would prove ineffective in the long term and suspected that eventually the vessel would reopen. However, proponents of VNUS Closure argued that so long as complete transmural cell death and fibrosis occurred across the entire length of the vein – as opposed to mere thrombus formation – very

1) Total Atrophy

2) Minor, non-significant patency

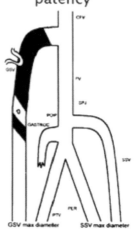

Figure 1.1: In the 11.1 year VNUS Closure trial, 68.6% of treated veins were fully closed and classified as a 'Category 1' success whilst 24.9% had near total closure of the treated vessel but for some minor patency of no clinical significance or the presence of some small vessels entering the GSV and were classified as 'Category 2' successes

3) Partial Failure, Refluxing Stump

4) Complete Re-opening

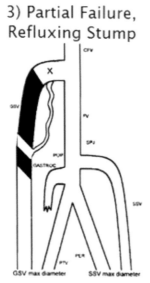
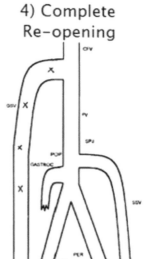

Figure 1.2: In the 11.1 year VNUS Closure trial, 5.9% of treated veins had a stump re-opening leading to clinically varicose veins and were classified as a 'Category 3' failure whilst 0.5% had complete patency in the treated vein and were classified as a 'Category 4' failure

good long term results should be expected[11].

In 2013, we reported a large scale clinical audit looking back at the results of VNUS Closure more than ten years after treatment[16]. The audit looked at 185 legs in 112 patients treated in our unit, which was the first unit in the United Kingdom to begin using VNUS Closure. At a mean of 11.1 years, it was seen that 93.5% of GSV treated with VNUS Closure remained successfully closed.

The treatment outcome was defined by the amount of vein atrophy at a mean of 11.1 years, as shown in Figure 1. Of the treated veins, 68.6% were completely closed and so were placed within the 1st category of success. 24.9% of veins had near complete atrophy, but either had minor patency of no clinical significance or the presence of minor veins and tributaries feeding into small portions of the former GSV, placing them within the 2nd Category of success (See Figure 1.1). In 11 legs (5.9%) there was a re-opening of a proximal, incompetent GSV stump which refluxed into clinical varicose veins, placing them within a failure score category of 3. In 1 case (0.5%), there was a complete re-opening of the treated vein placing it in failure category 4 (See Figure 1.2).

In line with studies carried out over shorter periods, the 11.1 year data showed no conventional SFJ neovascularization, apart from in 4 legs (2.2%) which had received traditional open varicose vein treatment at some point before the VNUS procedure. Within the trial, 7 primary legs (3.8%) did show the presence of some small vessels near the sapheno-femoral junction (SFJ) which had some similarity to neovascularization, despite that fact that VNUS Closure has previously been shown to avoid this[11]. However, it was seen on ultrasound that these small vessels were somewhat different in appearance to typical neovascularization and that similar patterns of connective tissue near the SFJ have been seen on ultrasound in legs which have never had vein treatment of any kind. Therefore, for the purposes of the trial the small SFJ vessels were not thought to represent neovascularization resulting from the VNUS Closure but a genetic form of serpentine veins. This may indeed be Primary Avalvular Varicose Anomalies (PAVA), a venous abnormality reported after this clinical audit took place[17].

VNUS Closure Failures

Of the small proportion of patients who experienced a failure of GSV closure in the long term VNUS trial, there were no particularly noteworthy demographic features. The age range for the group of failures at the time of the research scan was 36 to 86 (mean 65) versus 31 to 90 (mean 63) for the whole 112 patient group. The mean time between treatment and the research scan was 11.0 years for the failures and 11.1 for the whole group. The ratio of 7 female to 3 male patients (2.3:1) in the failure group was broadly similar to the 84 female to 28 male (3:1) patients seen for the entire data set. This indicates that there was no association between age or gender and the propensity for failure.

Despite the fact that 10 of the patients with failures had bilateral treatment, only 1 had a bilateral failure – indicating there was no significant association between genetic or environmental factors and the likelihood of a vein re-opening. All the patients who failed were treated in 2001 and 2002 – whereas the whole patient group was treated between 1999 and 2002. This may well indicate that more difficult patient cases were taken on as familiarity with the VNUS technique increased, or simply be due to the fact that 80/112 (71.4%) of the patients were treated in the latter two years. Whilst all the patients in the failure group were treated for primary (as opposed to recurrent) varicose veins at the time of the VNUS Closure, over 80% of patients within the trial, fit within this definition.

In 2001/2 when these treatments were carried out, duplex scanning and understanding of the venous system was not as advanced as it was in 2013 when this follow up audit was carried out. As such, some incompetent AASVs that were present before treatment may have been disguised by the siphon effect of a refluxing GSV and may have played a role in some of the GSV stump re-openings. Conversely though, in a number of these failures, the AASV had been successfully treated.

The non-genetic, non-environmental nature of the failures seen at a mean of 11.1 years, and the fact that even patients with large veins could receive a good result, suggests then that they may have been due to an error of technique. Since the introductory years of VNUS Closure, experience with endoluminal techniques has increased and modern thermoablation devices have improved and so it would be expected that failures of endovenous surgery resulting from technical errors would decrease in future.

Clinical Recurrence

Despite the fact that we found a very high success rate for the technique itself, a significant level of clinical recurrence of varicose veins was still seen (see Table 1). With the elimination of missed veins due to good ultrasound diagnosis and neovascularization due to thermoablation, by far the largest source of clinical recurrence at a mean of 11.1 years after VNUS Closure, was disease progression, with *de novo* reflux being seen in veins which had previously been competent at the time of treatment.

In 32.4% of legs in the trial, this *de novo* reflux took the form of incompetent major veins – AASV, SSV, perforator or pelvic veins – and in 14.6% of legs, less significant veins with no connection to the deep system. These latter veins were found to be refluxing and leading to varicose veins with a Clinical Etiology Anatomy Pathological classification (CEAP) clinical score of at least C2. In the future, the levels of 'non-truncal *de novo* reflux' which we have seen at a mean of 11.1 years following VNUS Closure may well be reduced, as the injection of foam sclerotherapy into minor veins during or following truncal vein surgery has now become common practice in ours and other specialist venous units.

It is possible that the level of truncal *de novo* reflux reported here may have been artificially high due to missing the siphon effect of GSV incompetence on some of the AASVs which may have been incompetent. Hence some of these could constitute 'missed' veins as opposed to *de novo* reflux.

It needs to be noted that this study, over decade after the original surgery, relied on patients agreeing to attend appointments for assessments and research scans, and paying themselves to travel the (often considerable) distance to the unit. These barriers would tend towards a negative feedback-bias. It therefore seems likely that the 112 patients who attended out of 359 who were invited (31.2%) would include a large proportion of those most concerned with the condition of their veins.

Whilst the factors above may have tended to increase the amount of clinical recurrence seen in

Cause of recurrence	Legs	Related to VNUS Surgery	May occur in other varicose vein treatment
Failure of the treatment	12 legs (6.5%)*,**	Yes	Yes
Small vessels at the SFJ	7 legs (3.8%)*	Possibly	Possibly
Neovascularization from previous surgery	4 legs (2.2%)*	No	Yes
De novo (truncal)	60 legs (32.4%)*	No	No
De novo (non-truncal) [sole cause of clinical reccurence]	27 legs (14.6%)*	No	No
Intermittent treatment (outside GSV) removed all clinical recurrence	11 legs (5.9%)		

Table 1: At a mean of 11.1 years following VNUS Closure, clinical recurrence of varicose veins was seen due to a variety of reasons. There were varicose veins arising from sources connected to the procedure itself, those coming from prior conventional surgery and finally disease progression.

(Red boxes denote clinical recurrence directly resulting from a failure of the VNUS procedure. Orange boxes denote clinical recurrence that may be a result of the VNUS procedure. Yellow boxes denote clinical recurrence directly resulting from treatment other than the VNUS procedure. Green boxes denote recurrence which would occur regardless of the treatment offered due to disease progression.)
*Some legs had multiple sources of clinical recurrence and so the same leg may appear in several categories
**Only those factors causing clinical recurrence at the 11.1 year audit were recorded, except for in the case of a Failure of the Treatment where all 12 failures over the whole time period were recorded, despite the fact that 3 of these had undergone further treatment in the interim and hence had been cured before the audit

this study, it is worth noting that a further subset of 11 legs (5.9%) had had intermittent treatment which removed all signs of varicose veins. Whilst intermittent treatment, which completely removed all clinical recurrence from a leg was easy to record, treatment which changed the causes of clinical recurrence (aside from that to the GSV) was not extensively investigated. Due to the fact that multiple components may contribute to recurrence and it is sometimes difficult to establish (especially retrospectively) if an individual factor would have independently caused clinical recurrence – only those factors causing varicose veins at the time of audit were recorded (with the exception of the GSV where intermittent failures were recorded even if they had subsequently been treated and were no-longer causing recurrence at review).

An issue also arises where a possible cause for recurrence was treated in one of these patients, before it was actually causing any clinically significant recurrent varicose veins. There may, for instance, have been more cases of small SFJ vessels which received intermittent foam sclerotherapy. Some of the legs classified as "*de novo* non-truncal reflux" may have had intermittent treatment which removed the *de novo* truncal reflux. At least 3 legs (1.6%) classified as "*de novo* non-truncal reflux" might have been classified as "*de novo* truncal reflux" were it not for intermittent treatment.

Of these 3 legs, 1 primary leg also contained neovascular type tissue in the fascia which the intermittent surgery removed. It would appear therefore that without minor intermittent treatment, small vessels at the SFJ might indeed have been a larger cause of recurrence. The "*de novo* non-truncal reflux" group also contained at least 4 legs (2.2%) which had had more minor intermittent treatment such as micro sclerotherapy, phlebotomies or in one case the SFJ excised, the effects of which were difficult to gauge. The factors which may have increased or decreased the amount of *de novo* reflux in the trial would seem to have broadly balanced out, as the overall rate of recurrence that we found agrees quite well with Brand et al. who showed that disease progression can be expected to arise at a rate of approximately 3% a year[18].

Patient and type of failure that developed in 11.1 year period	Treatment date	Scan date and vein status	Scan date and vein status	Time between treatment and scan
A Left partial failure	4/15/2002	2003: No Stump (but bifid segment with distal reflux)	2010: Stump open and refluxing	Approx.1 year and 8 years
B Right partial failure	11/05/2001	2006: No Stump	-	Approx. 5 years
C Left partial failure	3/26/2001	2007: No Stump	-	Approx. 6 years
D Left total failure	1/30/2001	2007: Total Failure	-	Approx. 6 years
E Left partial failure	04/02/2001	2007: Stump open and refluxing	2008: Stump open and refluxing after intermittent EVLA	Approx. 6 years
E Right partial failure	04/02/2001	2007: Stump open and refluxing	2008: No Stump after intermittent EVLA	Approx. 6 years

Table 2: Intermittent Scans on Failures
Of the 11 patients (12 legs) who had a GSV failure by 2012, from their VNUS Closure 2001/02, 5 (6 legs) had received duplex ultrasound scans in the intermittent period that remained readily available. These scans showed that 4 of the 6 of veins scanned between 5-8 years after treatment had already shown signs of re-opening. A 6th patient, (7th leg) had a refluxing GSV stump before undergoing intermittent EVLA to an incompetent lateral thigh vein along with foam sclerotherapy treatment approximately 6 years after initial treatment but the scan showing this could not be properly assessed.
Red boxes denote the first scan date which found re-opening in a treated GSV. Green boxes denote legs were the most recent scan before the review did not find any re-opening of the treated vein.

Of the 11 patients (12 legs) who had a partial or complete failure of the VNUS Closure at the time they were reviewed in 2012, 5 patients (representing 6 failures) had returned to the unit at some point since their treatment which had been carried out in 2001-2002 (see Table 2). Of these patients, 4 legs that would eventual fail were scanned in 2007 and 2 were found to already show a GSV stump and 1 (the only total failure in the review) was found to have already fully re-opened. The patient who had a complete re-opening of the vein in 1 leg had received bilateral VNUS treatment and interestingly, whilst his other leg showed a scarred, patent stump at approximately 6 years, none was recorded at the final scan, despite the fact that he had received no intermittent treatment. Whilst the 4th leg scanned in 2007 did not show a re-opening, stumps were not specifically looked for and so it may be that a very minor one was already present. A similar result to this was also seen in a patient scanned in 2006. The final patient was scanned in 2003 and did not have a record of a stump then, but one was visible at a re-scan in 2010.

In addition to these, 1 further patient had a refluxing GSV stump before receiving intermittent treatment – although the date of the diagnostic scan which diagnosed this could not be found. The data, whilst extremely limited, therefore shows that by 8 years, 4/6 (66.7%) of legs which would fail by the final scan at a mean of 11.1 years had already done so. From a theoretical point of view, it would seem unusual for many veins with full fibrosis to ever re-open and so it would have been useful if a detailed investigation specifically looking for very minor stumps could have been carried out on the two veins which had no recorded signs of failure at 5 and 6 years after treatment.

The results from this study with a mean review of 11.1 years post VNUS Closure suggests that if a treated vein remained closed all the way up to the SFJ with full fibrosis for a number of years then very few, if any, would be expected to ever go on to fail. This is in agreement with shorter term thermoablation data such as a study on results of EVLA by Sadick and Wasser which showed that the majority of re-openings seen at 4 years had occurred within 6 months of treatment and all of them within 12 months[19].

Conclusion

In many specialist venous centres endoluminal thermoablation has now become the standard course of treatment for incompetent truncal veins, followed or in association with, phlebectomy for large varices and foam sclerotherapy to smaller vessels. With long term results now showing good success rates for VNUS Closure, this trend is only expected to continue.

Thermoablation devices have now advanced beyond the first VNUS catheters, with several different techniques making use of mono-polar as opposed to bi-polar radiofrequency, laser ablation and steam. The far greater size of electrode in the new radiofrequency catheters and the increased energy provided by laser, means that the leg no longer needs to be compressed with bandaging and instead, a local anaesthetic can be injected around the vein to provide 'tumescence'. This protects the surrounding muscles and nerves from burning and also has the great advantage of abolishing the need for general anaesthetic.

Hence, thermoablation of veins has now become an office based, out-patient procedure. Despite these advances though, the techniques still works along the same principal as VNUS Closure: endoluminal thermoablation. So, whilst long term data is only available for a now obsolete technique, it produces the proof of concept to finally demonstrate the superiority of a lumen-delivered, fibrosis-inducing approach, over surgical stripping, at over ten years.

Since failures from VNUS Closure seem to be primarily based on an error in the technique and the devices used for endoluminal thermoablation have since improved significantly, it is therefore reasonable to expect that a similar unit, using modern thermoablation devices today, would see a better than 93.5% success rate in ablating the target truncal vein in 10 years' time.

References

1. Gaggiati, A; Allegra, C. (2006). Historical Introduction. In: Bergan, J The Vein Book. Burlington, MA, USA: Academic Press. 7.

2. Shami, S; Cheatle, T (2003). Fegan's Compression Sclerotherapy of Varicose Veins. 2nd ed. London, UK: Springer. 2003.

3. Madelung, O.W. Ueber die Ausschalung cirsoider Varicen an den Unteren Extremitatem. Verhandl Deutsch Gesellsch Chir. 1884; 13: 114-117

4. Keller, W.L. A new method of extirpating the internal saphenous and similar veins in varicose conditions: a preliminary report. N Y Med J. 1905; 82: 385

5. van Rij, AM; Jiang, P; Solomon, C; Christie, RA; Hill GB. (2003). Recurrence after varicose vein surgery: a prospective long-term clinical study with duplex ultrasound scanning and air plethysmography. Journal of Vascular Surgery. 38 (5), 935-943.

6. Jones L, Braithwaite BD, Selwyn D, Cooke S, Earnshaw JJ. Neovascularisation is the principle cause of varicose vein recurrence: results of a randomised trial of stripping the long saphenous vein. Eur J Vasc Endovasc Surg. 1996; 12(4): 442-5.

7. Campbell, WB; Vijay, Kumar A; Collin, TW; Allington, KL; Michaels, JA. (2003). The outcome of varicose vein surgery at 10 years: clinical findings, symptoms and patient satisfaction. Ann R Coll Surg Engl. 2003; 85(1): 52-57.

8. Smith, P. (2007). Ultrasound-Guided Foam Sclerotherapy for Chronic Venous Disease. In: Thompson, M; Morgan, R; Matsumura, J; Sapoval, M; Loftus, I Endovascular Intervention for Vascular Disease: Principles and Practice. New York, NY, USA: Informa Healthcare. 527.

9. Parsi K. Interaction of detergent sclerosants with cell membranes. Phlebology. 2015; 30: 306-15.

10. Morrison, N. VNUS Closure of the Saphenous Vein. In: Burgan, The Vein Book. Burlington, MA, USA: Academic Press. 2006. 283-284.

11. Whiteley MS, Holdstock JM. Percutaneous radiofrequency ablations of Varicose Veins (VNUS Closure). In: Vascular and Endovascular Challenges. Roger M Greenhalgh, editor. London; BIBA Publishing 2004. p 361- 381

12. Kianifard B, Holdstock JM, Whiteley MS. Radiofrequency ablation (VNUS closure) does not cause neo-vascularisation at the groin at one year: results of a case controlled study. Surgeon. 2006; 4 (2): 71-4.

13. Fassiadis N, Kianifard B, Holdstock JM, Whiteley MS. Ultrasound changes at the saphenofemoral junction and in the long saphenous vein during the first year of VNUS Closure. Int Angiol. 2002; 21 (3): 272-4.

14. Nicolini P, The Closure Group. Treatment of primary varicose veins by endovenous obliteration with the VNUS closure system: results of a prospective multicentre study. Eur J

Vasc Endovasc Surg. 2005; 29 (4): 433-9.

15. Merchant RF, Pichot O, The Closure Study Group. Long-term outcomes of endovenous radiofrequency obliteration of saphenous reflux as a treatment for superficial venous insufficiency. J Vasc Surg. 2005; 42 (3): 502-9.

16. Taylor DC, Whiteley AM, Fernandez-Hart TJ, Whiteley MS. Ten year results of radiofrequency ablation (VNUS Closure®) of the great saphenous and anterior accessory saphenous veins, in the treatment of varicose veins. Phlebology. 2013; 28 (6): 335

17. Ostler AE, Holdstock JM, Harrison CC, Fernandez-Hart TJ, Whiteley MS. Primary avalvular varicose anomalies are a naturally occurring phenomenon that might be misdiagnosed as neovascular tissue in recurrent varicose veins. J Vasc Surg Venous Lymphatic Disord. 2014; 2(4); 390-396.

18. Brand FN, Dannenberg AL, Abbott RD, Kannel WB. The epidemiology of varicose veins: the Framingham Study. Am J Prev Med. 1988; 4 (2): 96-101.

19. Sadick NS, Wasser S. Combined endovascular laser plus ambulatory phlebectomy for the treatment of superficial venous incompetence: A 4-year perspective . J Cosmet Laser Ther. 2007; 9(1): 9-13.

Chapter 5

Optimising the results of Radiofrequency-induced thermotherapy (RFiTT) – *in vitro, ex vivo* and clinical evidence to show how a new protocol was developed.

Author(s)
George E Badham[1]
Emma B Dabbs[1]
Mark S Whiteley[1,2]

Institution(s)
(1) The Whiteley Clinic, Stirling House, Stirling Road, Guildford, Surrey GU2 7RF
(2) Faculty of Health and Biomedical Sciences, University of Surrey, Guildford, Surrey GU2 7XH

Introduction

The introduction of minimally invasive endovenous surgery for the treatment of varicose veins and underlying venous reflux presented a new treatment option for patients. Traditional surgery was not only invasive and came with the added cost and risk of general or regional anaesthetic, but also caused pain, bruising, relatively large scarring and considerable time off work. In addition, open surgery is associated with recurrence due to neovascularisation[1], a problem that is not found in well-performed endovenous surgery[2].

Minimally invasive endovenous thermal ablation devices have largely eradicated the pain and bruising and should reduce the recurrence of varicose veins due to neovascularisation and strip-tract revascularisation observed with high saphenous ligation and stripping procedures[3].

Rather than the veins being surgically removed in open invasive and relatively traumatic procedures, the device is placed within the vein lumen and ablates the vein from the inside out. Initially the "closure" of the vein was attributed to collagen contraction. However, in 2004 we published our view that for a vein to be chronically occluded, transmural cell death across the vein wall must be achieved[4].

Endovenous radiofrequency ablation (RFA) was first performed in the UK by Mark Whiteley and Judy Holdstock on 12th March 1999, using the VNUS Closure® catheter. This device consisted of a central electrode surrounded by a second electrode, divided into four individual parts. An alternating current was passed between these two electrodes through the vein wall, oscillating at radiofrequency rates. This heated the vein wall to approximately 85°C. Consistent and sufficient heat was generated within the vein wall and evaluated through a continuous thermal feedback mechanism via a thermocouple on one of the electrodes, which was supposed to ensure that no damage was caused in surrounding tissue.

When thermal energy was passed into the vein wall, it appeared to "close". However, whether a vein is permanently "closed" or not after treatment depends on the pattern and the extent of damage inflicted on the vein wall and how the body responds to the pattern of the damage. If the thermal energy is insufficient to cause transmural death, or is given too quickly so that the inner part of the vein wall is over-treated and the outer part of the vein wall inadequately treated, thrombotic occlusion can occur. The living media leaves a living "vein skeleton" which, in combination with the intraluminal thrombosis, results in the possibility of "re-opening"[5].

Therefore, to achieve permanent ablation of the refluxing truncal vein with endothermal ablation devices, we believe it is essential to cause transmural death of the vein wall. To achieve this, an adequate amount of thermal energy is required, but this needs to be applied at a rate that allows conduction through the whole vein wall. We need to avoid applying energy too quickly, which can result in carbonisation on the inner surface and inadequate treatment of the outer layers.

RFiTT

Radiofrequency-induced thermotherapy (RFiTT) (Celon-Olympus Europa, Hamburg) is a catheter-based device that is used for endovenous thermoablation.

The RFiTT catheter has two circumferential electrodes at the tip, separated by a small gap. The RFiTT device is positioned by ultrasound and the patient is tipped into a head-down position. The position and the injection of tumescence around the vein causes contraction of the vein, ensuring that it is in contact with the electrodes. When the device is activated, an alternating current is passed between the two electrodes through the vein wall, at radiofrequency rates. Heat is generated by the resistance of the vein wall to the passage of the alternating current, and is not generated in the electrodes themselves. This mechanism is the same as in the original VNUS Closure® catheter. As RFiTT uses 2 electrodes, it is classified as bipolar radiofrequency ablation (Figure 1).

As with all catheter based thermoablation devices, RFiTT is introduced into the vein under ultrasound guidance using a Seldinger technique. Ultrasound is also used to position the tip prior to treatment and to guide tumescence.

Uniquely among the radiofrequency catheters, RFiTT monitors the impedance of the tissue to the passage of the electrical current. This is then converted into an audible pitch. The pitch is determined by the lowest impedance measured at the tip of the catheter. Once the vein is heated sufficiently it dries out (desiccates), which increases resistance to current flow (impedance) and consequently increases the tone of the pitch. When the tissue is completely dried and impedance reaches a certain threshold, the RFiTT generator cuts out automatically.

However, when the generator 'cuts out' it is not necessarily indicative of transmural vein damage. Although this feature is promoted as a signal to the desiccation of tissue and hence effectiveness of treatment, it is unclear as to the relative contributions of the amount of desiccation produced in

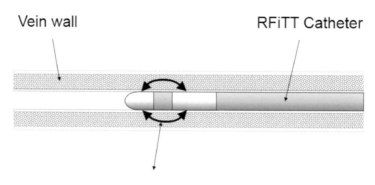

Vein wall   RFiTT Catheter

Passage of alternating electric
current through vein wall

Figure 1: A diagram of the RFiTT device inside a vein – it is a bipolar radiofrequency device that transmits a passage of alternating electric current through the vein wall between two electrodes.

tissue directly in contact with the electrodes (the intima) and the desiccation of the deeper levels of the vein wall (media and adventitia), particularly in veins of different wall thicknesses.

As we are aiming for transmural thermal ablation of the vein wall, this high impedance signal should not be used as a measure of transmural death and should not be used as the sole factor in deciding the rate of catheter withdrawal. Rather we would suggest that the energy input should be calculated and used as the guide for catheter withdrawal.

So How Much Energy Should Be Used?

There are two variables used to calculate how much energy is being applied to the vein wall.

These are:

- the energy the device is set at (measured in Watts or Joules per second J/s)
- the rate at which the device is withdrawn (in seconds per centimeter s/cm)*.

These two variables allow the Linear Endovenous Energy Density (LEED) to be calculated[6]. The LEED is a measure of the total energy being emitted over the length of vein being treated and so it is measured in J/cm.

The LEED is very important as previous studies looking at the results of the treatment of veins by thermoablation devices have only shown good levels of closure using a LEED greater than 60 J/cm, both in RFiTT[7] and Endovenous Laser Therapy[8]. Increasing the LEED with endovenous radiofrequency ablation devices does not seem to lead to higher postoperative pain[7].

---

* Whilst speed is defined as distance / time and hence measured in cm/s, we have found it more useful to quantify the withdrawal of the catheter in s/cm. This is because it is a practical measure during treatment. It is logical to monitor the cm marks on the catheter as it is being withdrawn, and to alter the speed of withdrawal depending on how many seconds are passing.

Early RFiTT Results And Clinical Problems

When the RFiTT device was first introduced, questions were raised about what exact rate of pull-back and power level that the device should be set at to achieve good results. In the past, *ex vivo* experiments[9] and clinical trials[10] have favored high-power RFiTT levels between 18 and 25 W with withdrawal rates of approximately 1s/cm, giving a LEED in the region of only 20 J/cm.

Indeed, a LEED of 20 J/cm was the initial recommendation with a power of 20 W and a pullback of 1 s/cm. The justification for this seems to have come from previous generations of the technology used in other areas of medicine such as tumor ablation.[11]

Despite this being a "recommendation", reports from units using less than 60 J/cm for endovascular procedures included: early re-openings (the vein becoming patent and refluxing after initially looking as if they had been successfully "closed" on duplex ultrasound), "sticking" and high-impedance cutting out[7]. Sticking of the catheter occurs when the catheter tip becomes adherent to the vein wall during treatment due to burnt (carbonized) tissue on the electrodes, interrupting smooth and continuous pullback. This presented practical problems for the doctor making effective treatment difficult to deliver, as this often necessitated frequent catheter removal for cleaning the burnt debris off of the electrodes.

Catheter sticking and the RFiTT generator cutting out due to high impedance made it very difficult to perform a smooth continuous pullback. Catheter sticking was also uncomfortable for some patients, despite tumescent anaesthesia, as the patients are aware of a tugging sensation when the tip is pulled free of the charred tissue.

Our Thoughts About These Initial Problems

When using 18 or 20 W, the tissue in contact with the electrodes was heated, but we felt that the power was being delivered too rapidly to allow the thermal energy to be conducted effectively through the remaining vein wall. Hence, we felt that the sticking of the device and the high impedance cut-outs of the system during treatments, coupled with the carbon found on the electrodes when the device was removed, showed that the power level was too high. As the total LEED was low (20 J/cm if 20 W power was used with a 1s/cm pullback) then there would not be enough total power to cause transmural death. Logically this would mean that the energy was being wasted on the innermost layer of the vein wall whilst leaving the media and adventitia inadequately treated.

Carbonization greatly limits the therapeutic efficacy of thermoablation. Carbonized tissue will increase impedance initiating the RFiTT cut off, stopping the spread of thermal energy deeper into the vein wall. Consequently, the "vein skeleton" of living media and adventitia surrounding this carbonized tissue remains healthy, which, as we described in 2005, is likely to result in recanalisation in the future.[12]

The carbonized tissue in the inner layers of the vein are highly thrombogenic. So as the device is withdrawn, any blood entering the "treated" section of the vein will thrombose. On colour duplex ultrasonography, such intraluminal thrombus is reported as successful "closure" of the vein, as the thrombus prevents any flow within the vein lumen. Unfortunately, thrombus contains many pro-endothelial stem cells and so, during the healing process, it is easy to hypothesize that the carbonized tissue is removed by the cellular immune system, the thrombus develops re-vascularization channels as is seen after stripping with strip tract re-vascularization[3]. These new (incompetent) vein channels coalesce into a new lumen, supported by the living media and adventitia of the "vein skeleton".

Thus, we believe that techniques or protocols reporting early "closure" with subsequent "re-opening" of the section of vein that was "treated", were actually failures from the beginning that had been erroneously reported as early "closures" due to the formation of intraluminal thrombus rather than closure by ablation of the vein wall and transmural death leading to subsequent atrophy.

Overall, when a LEED less than 60 J/cm is used during thermoablation of an average incompetent Great Saphenous Vein (GSV), there is a risk of destruction of the intima alone leading to sticking, carbonization, luminal thrombus, recanalization, re-opening and subsequent failure of closure.[7,8,11]

Developing A New Protocol

It was clear to us that a LEED greater than 60 J/cm was crucial to the success of endovenous ablation with the RFiTT device. Therefore, we set up a study which aimed to develop a reproducible method of using RFiTT where the LEED produced was greater than 60 J/cm but did not cause sticking, carbonization or high impedance cut outs.

Theoretically, there were two ways to achieve this. We could increase the power setting of the device meaning more energy was being applied to the vein wall over each centimeter. Alternatively, we could slow down the pullback of the device, allowing a lower power setting to have more time to apply energy to the vein wall for each centimeter of pull back.

As carbonization and sticking were already a problem with the RFiTT device when it was used at high power settings, it was clear to us that we would need to reduce the power and slow down the pull back, allowing heat to conduct away from the device and spread within the vein wall, attaining our minimum target LEED of 60 J/cm, ensuring transmural death and successful vein wall thermoablation whilst avoiding carbonization by over-treating the intima.

In-Vitro Model – Porcine Liver

To measure the effect of different combinations of power and pullback speeds, we designed an *in vitro* experiment. This involved using porcine liver as a model for biological tissue to be ablated (ie: a model for thermal ablation into the vein wall) under a glass plate. The glass allowed measurements, pictures and videos to be taken showing the effects of the thermocoagulation of the liver tissue by the RFiTT device.

Porcine liver was chosen for 3 main reasons. Firstly, liver has a similar cell density to that found in human veins. Secondly, there is a precedent to using liver models in radiofrequency devices used in other medical settings[13]. Thirdly, porcine liver is dark when raw but goes light when the tissue is heated sufficiently to coagulate proteins. We took this to be representative of successful thermal ablation for two reasons. Firstly, cells which have been heated sufficiently to have had their constituent proteins coagulated are dead. Secondly, protein coagulation causes contraction which is the second element of venous closure in thermal ablation (see Chapter 1: Endovenous thermal ablation of varicose veins and examination of the use and failings of linear endovenous energy density (LEED) by Mark Whiteley).

Using this model, we needed to identify a surrogate "end-point" which would represent successful transmural thermal ablation in a vein wall. In order to do this, it was essential to determine how far the thermal ablative effect should spread laterally (or perpendicularly to the axis of the device) from the device. Studies of the thickness of the great saphenous vein wall have found it to be highly variable, with thicknesses between 0.18 and 0.65mm.[14] As we were developing a protocol to fit most Great Saphenous Veins, a 'worst case scenario' approach was taken and the vein wall assumed to be 0.65mm in thickness. Therefore, a thermal spread of greater than 0.65mm was taken as necessary to effectively treat a standard incompetent Great Saphenous Vein.

The results of these *in vitro* experiments using a porcine liver model have been published in a peer-reviewed journal.[15]

Results

Carbonization, sticking and impedance cut-outs

When we used the previously recommended settings - high powers of 18 W or 20 W and a pull-back speed withdrawing the catheter at 1 s/cm - inadequate thermoablation was found in this model using the criteria that we had decided upon (Figure 2). This is not surprising as we have seen above, even a power of 20 W will only produce a LEED of 20 J/cm with this fast pull-back. A LEED of 20 J/cm is known to be inadequate for successful and reproducible thermoablation of GSVs. As such, the results from our model would seem to be in keeping with what we know clinically.

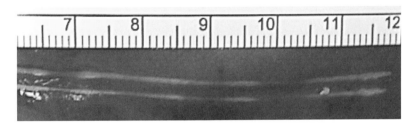

Figure 2: Porcine liver model with RFiTT treatment using 20 W at 1 s/cm pullback (LEED of 20 J/cm), showing inadequate treatment.

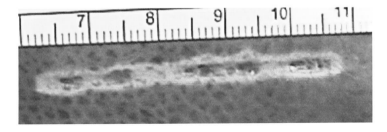

Figure 3: Porcine liver model with RFiTT treatment using 20 W at 5 s/cm (LEED of 100 J/cm), showing carbonization.

When the pull-back was slowed to 3 s/cm with the same power (to attain a LEED of 60 J/cm) carbonization of the liver and sticking of the tip to the tissue was found, mirroring what is found when these settings are used to attempt ablation in incompetent truncal veins. Furthermore, slowing the pull-back speed further to 5 s/cm (to obtain a LEED of 100 J/cm) produced what we considered to be an unacceptable level of carbonization, with almost continuous high impedance cut-outs during the pull-back (Figure 3).

Overall, whenever 18 or 20 W were used, either the pull-back speed had to be fast in which case the LEED was too low, or if it was slowed sufficiently to get the LEED higher than 60 J/cm, carbonization, sticking and impedance cut-outs were observed.

Conversely when the power was dropped to 12 W or less, and pull-back speed were slowed to achieve LEEDs of 72 J/cm, carbonization, sticking, or impedance cut-outs reduced significantly and indeed were not found in any experiment with power levels of 6W.

Thermal spread

The thermal spread was measured by taking the digital image of the treated section of liver, magnifying it maximally and then counting the pixels from the edge where the device had sat, to the point where the ablated liver changed color back to non-treated liver, measured perpendicular to the axis of the device, or just "laterally". As each image included a ruler, the number of pixels making up 1 mm on the ruler could be checked for each image, giving a standardization of the measurements. The thermal spread at each of the settings tested are shown in the graph in Figure 4.

When a LEED of 18 or 20 J/cm was applied, thermal energy spread less than 0.5mm lateral from the device. Taking into consideration our chosen minimum of vein thickness of 0.65mm, this is not sufficient for deep thermal penetration and adequate vein wall damage.

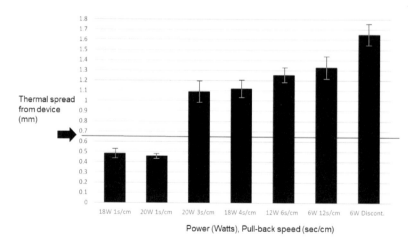

Figure 4: A graph to show the mean thermal spread at each tested setting. The arrow and corresponding line across the graph is at 0.65 mm, the chosen value of maximum wall thickness. Only LEED >60 J/cm reached a thermal spread over the desired value.

66

All LEEDs over 60 J/cm, regardless of which power and pull-back were used, showed thermal spread over 1mm lateral from the device.

However, these results show a progression of lateral thermal spread with slower pull-back speeds having a larger thermal spread, even if lower powers are used.

The 12 W at 6 s/cm and 6 W at 12 s/cm (Figure 5), both of which give a LEED of 72 J/cm, did not show any significant difference of thermal spread. However, applying a discontinuous pullback (6 sec at 6 W, then pullback 0.5 mm and repeat - giving a LEED of 72 J/cm) produced a mean thermal spread of 1.66mm (Figure 6), which was significantly higher than any other settings tested. In all cases when these lower powers were used, no carbonization or impedance cut-outs were observed.

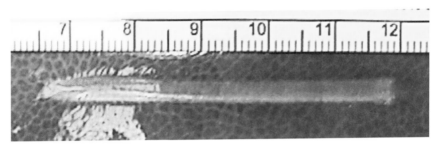

Figure 5: Porcine liver model with RFiTT treatment using 6 W at 12 s/cm pullback (LEED of 72 J/cm).

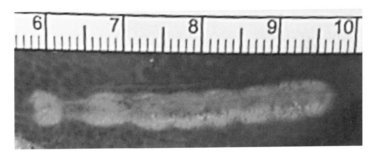

Figure 6: Porcine liver model with RFiTT treatment using discontinuous pullback of 6W at 6 seconds, then pullback 0.5 mm and repeat (LEED of 72 J/cm), showing a significantly higher thermal spread than any other setting.

Hence, from this work, we concluded that in this model, the optimal protocol for RFiTT treatment of a GSV would be a power of 6W and a discontinuous pull-back of holding the device stationary for 6 seconds, pulling it back for 5mm and then repeating and so on. This would give a thermal energy of 36 J per 0.5cm or a LEED of 72 J/cm.

From Porcine Liver to *Ex-Vivo* Great Saphenous Vein
While our porcine model allowed us to analyse several aspects of the thermal damage of biological

tissue using RFiTT, it still has some limitations due to it being an *in vitro* model. Two of the most obvious limitations were: firstly, the RFiTT device was placed on the liver under a piece of glass, and therefore was not completely surrounded by biological tissue as it would be *in vivo*; and secondly, whilst porcine liver is a good model, it is of course not identical to vein tissue.

Therefore, it was necessary to check if the results obtained in the porcine liver model translated into the same, or similar, findings when applied to the GSV itself. Such a correlation was necessary to justify the clinical application of the new protocol that the porcine liver model had suggested as optimal.

These results have also been published in a peer-reviewed journal, in a separate paper from the original porcine liver work.[16]

In this study, we used an incompetent GSV, harvested from a volunteer during varicose vein surgery. The explanted GSV was treated *ex vivo* with the following conditions:

1. One section left untreated as a control
2. 18 W with 1 s/cm pullback (LEED 18 J/cm)
3. 20 W with 1 s/cm pullback (LEED 20 J/cm)
4. 18 W with 3 s/cm pullback (LEED 54 J/cm)
5. 6 W with discontinuous 12s/cm pullback (LEED 72 J/cm)

Results from this *ex vivo* investigation correlated quite closely with those obtained from the *in vitro* porcine model. When administering a LEED of 18 or 20 J/cm, thermal damage was only really observed in the intima, with minimal damage to the media in the GSV, and in the porcine liver model a maximum thermal ablation measurement was found to be 0.5 mm with both energy levels. Hence, both *ex vivo* vein and porcine liver models agreed this is a sub-optimal result.

When the *ex vivo* GSV was treated at 18W with a LEED of 54 J/cm, the catheter adhered to the inner surface of the vein, suggesting some tissue carbonization and, in addition, high-impedance cut-outs occurred. The histology of the GSV showed ablation of the intima and media, and the inner half of the adventitia, a measured depth of 0.9mm. This correlated well with the porcine liver model that showed a good thermal spread in the liver as a mean of 1.09mm was measured.

As such, both *ex vivo* GSV and porcine liver models show that the thermal spread is adequate for transmural death and hence successful thermoablation. However, both also show a tendency for carbonization of the intima, device sticking and high impedance cut-outs. Hence, both models show this setting to be sub-optimal in terms of catheter sticking and intimal carbonization.

Finally, using a power of 6W and a discontinuous pullback of 6 seconds per 0.5mm giving a LEED of 72 J/cm, no catheter sticking, no carbonization nor high impedance cut-outs were observed. The GSV histology showed thermal ablation in all three layers of the vein wall, correlating well with the porcine liver model which showed a mean thermal spread measured at 1.65mm.

With the good correlation between the *in vitro* porcine liver model and the *ex vivo* GSV study, and in view of the poor clinical results reported in published papers using 18W and 20W (with both failures of ablation and the need to remove the device to clean the carbon debris off of the electrodes) we decided to adopt the new 6W discontinuous protocol as our standard treatment for RFiTT ablation of the GSV and other truncal veins.

Clinical evidence

Having implemented our new RFiTT protocol on laboratory based evidence, we felt it important to audit the results that we then obtained when using it in patients clinically.

Sixty three patients underwent RFiTT treatment of their incompetent GSV, small saphenous vein (SSV) and/or anterior accessory saphenous vein (AASV) using The Whiteley Clinic RFiTT protocol. They were all invited back as part of a 1 year audit, during which they were examined and a duplex ultrasound scan of the treated vein was performed.

Thirty five patients returned and the mean follow-up from treatment to audit scan was 16.3 months. There were 48 legs included with 64 truncal veins treated (34 GSV, 15 SSV and 15 AASV). Every one of the treated veins was found to be undergoing atrophy with no sign of any flow at all in any treated segment. Although some clinicians report "closure" of veins, we feel it is important to draw a distinction between atrophy which is likely to be permanent and "closed" which might merely represent a thrombosed vein which might re-canalise in the future.

These results were published with the full explanation in 2017[17].

The Whiteley Clinic Protocol for RFiTT thermoablation

Our protocol using 6W and a discontinuous pull-back of 6 seconds ablation then pulling back 0.5 mm and repeating the 6 seconds ablation and so on, achieves several important goals:

1. A LEED of 72 J/cm.
2. Virtually no carbonization making sticking and cut-outs rare.
3. A simple pull-back technique that is easily reproducible and can be taught easily rather than trying to get a smooth pull-back at a certain exact rate.
4. Laboratory proof of efficacy showing thermal spread of >0.65 mm in the porcine liver model and transmural thermal ablation in the GSV.
5. A clinical audit showing efficacy in ablating incompetent truncal veins.

Conclusion

Endovenous catheter based thermoablation has many advantages over open surgery for venous reflux and varicose veins and is now the recommended primary treatment for symptomatic varicose veins of truncal origin in the UK[18].

RFiTT is a bipolar radiofrequency ablation device designed for endovenous thermoablation. However, the recommended power levels for RFiTT treatments of truncal veins of 18W or 20W have resulted in the catheter sticking during treatment, carbonization of the tissue necessitating withdrawal of the catheter from the patient for cleaning of the treatment tip, high impedance cut-outs by the RFiTT generator, low LEEDs and failures of closure.

We have developed "The Whiteley Clinic Protocol for RFiTT" treatment of truncal incompetent veins that corrects all of these problems. We explored the problem using a porcine liver model to understand the thermal effects of RFiTT on biological tissue and from that, developed the protocol. We then showed that this work was reproducible in *ex vivo* GSV. This made us change our clinical protocol and a subsequent clinical audit showed that the protocol was 100% effective when used in patients.

We believe that this process of understanding the interaction of endovenous treatments with biological tissue and the development of optimized protocols is possible before starting clinical studies and would save some patients undergoing sub-optimal results. We have now introduced this as a standard process using these and more sophisticated models, to investigate all endovenous treatments both thermal and non-thermal.

Acknowledgements

The authors would like to thank Simon Ford of Olympus who started experimenting with different power levels in an *in vitro* model and shared his early results.

References

1. Jones L, Braithwaite BD, Selwyn D, Cooke S, Earnshaw JJ. Neovascularisation is the principal cause of varicose vein recurrence: results of a randomised trial of stripping the long saphenous vein. Eur J Vasc Endovasc Surg. 1996; 12(4): 442-5.

2. Kianifard B, Holdstock JM, Whiteley MS. Radiofrequency ablation (VNUS Closure®) does not cause neo-vascularisation at the groin at one year: Results of a case controlled study. Surgeon. 2006; 4(2); 71-4

3. Munasinghe A, Smith C, Kianifard B, Price BA, Holdstock JM, Whiteley MS Strip-track revascularization after stripping of the great saphenous vein. Br J Surg. 2007; 94 (7): 840-3

4. Whiteley MS, Holdstock JM. Percutaneous radiofrequency ablations of Varicose Veins (VNUS Closure). In: Vascular and Endovascular Challenges. Roger M Greenhalgh, editor. London; BIBA Publishing 2004. p 361- 381

5. New Methods of Vein Ablation. Mark Whiteley. In: Venous Disease Simplified Eds: Alun H Davies, Tim Lees & Ian F Lane. UK: Harley 2006

6. Proebstle TM, Krummenauer F, Gul D, et al. Nonocclusion and early reopening of the great saphenous vein after endovenous laser treatment is fluence dependent. Dermatol Surg. 2004; 30: 174–178.

7. Boon R, Akkersdijk GJM, Nio D. Percutaneus treatment of varicose veins with bipolar radiofrequency ablation. Eur J Radiol. 2010; 75(1): 43-47

8. Proebstle TM, Moehler T, Gül D, Herdemann S. Endovenous Treatment of the Great Saphenous Vein Using a 1,320 nm Nd:YAG Laser Causes Fewer Side Effects than Using a 940 nm Diode Laser. Dermatol Surg. 2005; 31: 1678–1684.

9. Reich-Schupke S1, Mumme A and Stucker M. Histopathological findings in varicose veins following bipolar radiofrequency-induced thermotherapy–results of an *ex vivo* experiment. Phlebology. 2011; 26: 69–74.

10. Braithwaite B, Hnatek L, Zierau U, et al. Radiofrequency-induced thermal therapy: results

of a European multicentre study of resistive ablation of incompetent truncal varicose veins. Phlebology. 2013; 28: 38–46.

11. Häcker A, Vallo S, Weiss C, et al. Technical characterization of a new bipolar and multipolar radiofrequency device for minimally invasive treatment of renal tumors. BJU Int. 2006; 97(4): 822–828

12. Whiteley MS. Varicose veins: endovascular options.. In: Roger M Greenhalgh ed, Towards Vascular and Endovascular Consensus. London; Biba Publishing 2005. p 564 – 572

13. Zurbuchen U, Frericks B, Roggan A, Lehmann K, Bossenroth D, et al. Ex Vivio Evaluation of a Biploar Application Concept for Radiofrequency Ablation. Anticancer Res. 2009; 29(4): 1309-14.

14. Canham PB, Finlay HM, Toughener DR. Contrasting structure of the saphenous vein and internal mammary artery used as coronary bypass vessels. Cardiovascular Res. 1997; 34: 557–56

15. Badham GE, Strong SM, Whiteley MS. An *in vitro* study to optimize treatment of varicose veins with radiofrequency-induced thermos therapy. Phlebology. 2015; 30 (1): 17-23

16. Badham GE, Dos Santos SJ, Whiteley MS. Radiofrequency induced thermotherapy (RFiTT) in a porcine liver model and *ex vivo* great saphenous vein. Minim Invasive Ther Allied Technol. 2017; 2: 1-7.

17. Badham GE, Dos Santos SJ, Lloyd LBA, Holdstock JM, Whitetely MS. One-year results of the use of endovenous radiofrequency ablation utilising an optimised radiofrequency-induced thermotherapy protocol for the treatment of truncal superficial venous reflux. Phlebology. DOI: 10.1177/0268355517696611

18. NICE (National Institute for Health and Care Excellence) clinical guidelines - CG 168. Varicose veins in the legs: the diagnosis and management of varicose veins. Issued: July 2013. http://publications.nice.org.uk/varicose-veins-in-the-legs-cg168

Chapter 6

Outcomes of EVLA – variation between different wavelengths and between bare-tipped and jacket tipped fibres

Author
Athanasios Vlahos

Institution
Vascular & Interventional Radiology, 911 N. Elm Street, Suite 128, Hinsdale, Illinois 60521

The concept of thermal ablation brought us two advanced technologies for the treatment of chronic venous insufficiency. Radiofrequency ablation and endovenous laser ablation were introduced in the late 1990's as viable alternatives to stripping the great and short saphenous veins. While both technologies are highly effective at closure, post-operative pain and bruising are still a concern. In this chapter, we will focus on endovenous laser ablation and try to answer the questions: Does wavelength have an effect on closure rates and post-operative side effects? And do jacket tipped fibres improve post-operative outcomes?

Initially, investigators of EVLA theorized that direct contact with the vessel wall was an important mechanism of action for closure[1, 2]. They relied upon pulsed energy with manual compression in their initial studies. This resulted in numerous perforations at the contact site between the bare tip fibre and the vessel wall causing a high rate of pain and bruising. In well-known studies by Proebstle[3] and Perkowski[4], it was determined that the primary mechanism of action of EVLA was the formation of steam bubbles created by the energy of the laser. The steam bubbles, in turn, create enough thermal injury to the vein endothelium, that thrombotic occlusion occurs[3, 4]. The areas where the bare tip actually touched the vein wall, resulted in perforation and extravasation resulting in an increased incidence of pain and bruising. Proebstle[5] went on to evaluate specific laser wavelengths, specifically, the 810, 940 and 980-nm wavelengths. In an *in vitro* generator of steam bubbles, he found that these wavelengths did not generate steam bubbles in plasma or saline alone, but rather in haemolytic blood[5]. These findings indicated that haemoglobin played an integral part in steam bubble formation. The 810, 940, 980, and the 1064-nm wavelengths became known as haemoglobin specific wavelengths.

Linear endovenous energy density (LEED), simply defined as joules per centimetre delivered to the vein, and power (Watts) have also been evaluated in the past for their influence on treatment outcomes. Studies in the past have shown that the optimal LEED range for lasers ranges from 60 J/cm to 100 J/cm [5,6]. Closure rates do improve somewhat with a LEED> 100J/cm with 100% success rates quoted in the past, however, the rate of paraesthesia was markedly higher in limbs that received a LEED >100J/cm (15.5%), compared to limbs that received <100 J/cm (2.3%) [7]. Power (Watts) has been investigated in the past to see if it had any influence on treatment outcomes. In a study using a 1470nm laser at 15W and 25W settings, with average LEEDs of 109.7 J/cm and 132.6 J/cm respectively, no statistically significant difference in efficacy or side effects was observed[8]. However, investigators observed a lower instance of bruising and reduced use of analgesics in the 15W group.

Given all of the above, investigators have examined the effects of different wavelengths on closure rates and side effects. One of the earliest studies on the subject compared an 810nm laser to a 980nm laser. Closure rates were similar in both groups, but the 980nm group demonstrated considerably less bruising (P<.005) at one-week post-procedure as well as lower pain (P<.05) at 4 months[9]. Recently 1320 and 1470-nm lasers have entered the endovenous market. These are commonly referred to as the water-specific laser wavelengths (WSLWs) [10, 11]. It is theorized that they cause vein wall damage by targeting the interstitial fluid in the vein wall. The 1320 and 1470-nm lasers are thought to behave in this fashion, having a higher affinity for water.

Studies examining longer wavelengths have also been performed. One study compared an 810nm laser with a 1320nm laser[10]. This was performed only in patients with bilateral venous insufficiency so both lasers could be used in the same patient. The same treatment parameters of 8W and a target LEED of 80 J/cm were employed. Ecchymosis and pain were examined in both treatment groups. At 3-4 days post procedure, ecchymosis and pain were less in the 1320nm treated group, however, formal statistical analysis was not performed. This suggested that the higher wavelength is a contributing factor to less side effects[10]. A study performed by Almeida et al.[11] compared the 1470nm laser to the 980nm laser. The 980nm laser group functioned as the control, with 14 limbs treated at a power setting of 12W and a target LEED of 80 J/cm. Another 41 limbs were treated with the 1470nm laser with power and energy settings ranging from 3W with a LEED of 20 J/cm to 5W with a LEED of 30 J/cm[11]. At 1 month follow up, both groups demonstrated 100% closure rates. A 10-point scale was used to assess pain. The treatment length where bruising was visible was used to measure ecchymosis. The 1470nm group reported a pain score of 0 in all cases. The 980nm reported a pain score of 1.9 (P<.0020). Based on the percentage of the treatment length that showed bruising, 79% of the 980nm group experienced moderate (25-49% of treatment length) or severe (50-100% of treatment length) bruising[11]. The 1470nm group demonstrated 10% moderate to severe bruising. Since a much lower wattage setting was used in the 1470nm group, it is difficult to separate the effects of less power or higher wavelength on bruising and ecchymosis.

Investigators have examined the effects of bare tipped fibres versus jacket tip fibres. The idea is that despite our best efforts, bare tip contact with the vessel wall is both unpredictable and unavoidable. This contact with vessel wall can lead to vessel perforation and extravasation, thus increasing bruising and pain. The theory behind jacket tipped, or covered fibres, is that by encasing the energy-emanating portion of the laser fibre, the emitting face of the bare tipped fibre will not make contact with the vessel wall.

One such fibre, (NeverTouch, AngioDynamics Inc., Queensbury, NY) was evaluated in a randomized study[12]. The covered fibre is a metallic-tip, secured onto a 600-micron optical fibre using a weld, which causes a divergence of laser "light" [13]. This divergence actually increases the effective fibre diameter to 905 microns. This, in turn, produces power density at a rate that is 2.2 times lower than bare tipped fibres, leading to 56% less power interaction with blood[13]. This generates coagulation as opposed to a cutting action experienced with bare tipped fibres. This allows the metallic tip fibre to generate high LEEDs using significantly less wattage. The metallic tip design also provides a 0.010" buffer between the emanating portion of the fibre and the vein wall[13].

In the study, patients were randomized into the RF, bare tip or covered-tip group. Standard RFA protocols were used in the RF group. The protocol used for the laser groups with continuous pullback of each fibre at a target energy rate of 100 J/cm at 12W with a 980nm laser[12]. At 72 hours, 100% closure was demonstrated in all groups. A 10-point analogue pain scale was used and patients were asked to record their pain scores each day, for seven days. At 7 days, a nurse who was blinded to fibre use graded each patient's ecchymosis using a scale of 0-5. The covered tip group reported an average pain score of 0.96, comparable to RF (0.80) and less than the bare tipped group (1.87). The average bruise score was 1.21 for the covered tip group, 1.45 for the bare tip group and 1.34 for the RF group. The relatively small group of patients in the covered group (10) makes it difficult to establish concrete conclusions, however, the study does add evidence that there is no need for laser-tip wall contact to ablate the vein.

Endothermal ablation, whether RF or laser, has become a viable and often superior option over the widely used vein stripping methods. Post-operative pain and bruising are still issues and have stimulated continued research in improving these technologies. The introduction of higher wavelengths have given us options in reducing pain and bruising. The jacket tip fibre study does provide early evidence that by eliminating fibre contact with the vein wall, it not only provides a more efficient way of delivering laser energy, but also it eliminates vessel perforation, leading to less pain and bruising. Hopefully, this pilot study will generate further investigations with jacket-tip fibres in order to solidify these claims.

References

1. Kabnick, Lowell S. Venous Laser Update: New Fibers Decrease power Density Smoothing Post Operative Recovery.

2. Min RJ, Zimmet SE, Isaacs MN, Forrestal MD. Endovenous Laser Treatment of the incompetent Greater Saphenous Vein. J Vasc Interv Radiol. 2001; 12: 1167-1171.

3. Proebstle TM, Lehr HA, Kargl A, et al. Endovenous treatment of the greater saphenous vein with a 940nm diode laser: thrombotic occlusion after thermal damage by laser-generated steam bubbles. J Vasc Surg. 2002; 35: 729-736.

4. Perkowski P, Ravi R, Gowda RCN. Endovenous Laser Ablation of the Saphenous Vein for Treatment of Venous Insufficiency and Varicose Veins.: Early Results From a Large Single-

Center experience. J Endovasc Ther. 2004; 11: 132-138.

5. Proebstle TM, Sandhofer M, Kargyl A, et al. Thermal Damage of the Inner Vein Wall During Endovenous Laser Treatment: Key Role of Energy Absorption by intravascular Blood. Dermatol Surg. 2002; 28: 596-600.

6. Theivacumar NS, Dellagrammaticas D, Beale RJ, et al. Factors influencing the Effectiveness of Endovenous Laser Ablation (EVLA) in the Treatment of Great Saphenous Vein Reflux. Eur J Vasc Endovasc Surg. 2008; 35: 119-123.

7. Pannier F, Rabe E, Maurins U. First results with a new 1470-nm diode laser for endovenous ablation of incompetent saphenous veins. Phlebology. 2009; 24: 26-30.

8. Maurins U, Rabe E, Pannier F. Does laser power influence the results of endovenous laser ablation (EVLA) of incompetent saphenous veins with the 1470-nm diode laser? A prospective randomized study comparing 15 and 25W. Int Angiol. 2009;28(1): 32-37.

9. Kabnick, L. Outcome of different endovenous laser wavelengths for great saphenous vein ablation. J Vasc Surg. 2006;43(1): 88-93.

10. Mackay EG, Almeida JI, Raines JK. Do different laser wavelengths translate into different patient outcomes? Endovascular Today. 2006: 45-48.

11. Almeida J, Mackay E., Javier J et al. Saphenous Laser Ablation at 1470 nm Targets the Vein Wall, Not Blood. Vasc Endovasc Surg. 2009; 43(5): 467-472.

12. Kabnick LS. Jacket-Tip Laser Fiber vs. Bare-Tip Laser fiber for Endothermal Venous Ablation of the Great Saphenous Vein: Are the Results the Same? Presented at: Controversies in and Updates Vascular Surgery; January 2008; Paris.

13. AngioDynamics. 2009. NeverTouch Power Density. Queensbury: AngioDynamics.

Chapter 7

The Bubble Trap Technique

Author(s)
Emma B Dabbs[1]
Tim J Fernandez-Hart[1]
Mark S Whiteley[1,2]

Institution(s)
(1) The Whiteley Clinic, Stirling House, Stirling Road, Guildford, Surrey GU2 7RF
(2) Faculty of Health and Biomedical Sciences, University of Surrey, Guildford, Surrey GU2 7XH

Introduction

Since the late 1990's the use of traditional surgery for the treatment of truncal venous reflux and varicose veins has been largely overtaken by minimally invasive catheter-based techniques. Rather than removing the incompetent vein in an invasive procedure, minimally invasive endovenous thermal ablation techniques destroy the cells of the vein wall in such a way that subsequently activates the body's immune system to remove the dead cells, causing fibrosis of the vein and achieving long-term reflux cessation. Endovenous thermal ablation devices have revolutionised venous surgery; the success rates are at least as good as those of stripping, and varicose vein surgery is now no longer associated with the high long-term surgical failure rate due to new vessel formation[1-3].

Minimally invasive thermal ablation devices initially treated the vein using radiofrequency with the advent of the VNUS Closure® catheter in 1998. Using this device, resistance to the passage of an alternating current at radiofrequency rates, passed between 2 electrodes through the vein wall, caused contraction of the proteins in the vein wall and heat-induced cell death. It was previously believed that the advantage of using thermal ablation was that, due to being minimally invasive, the procedure itself was less invasive and therefore less painful, resulting in fewer side-effects and allowed faster return to work[4-6]. However, it soon became clear that ablating the vein with heat energy rather than removing it in traumatic procedures provided many more long-term benefits. The biggest advantage of endovenous thermal ablation for the treatment of truncal venous reflux is that it does not cause neovascularisation in the groin, which is the most common cause of recurrent varicose veins after stripping[3,7].

It was previously believed that during endovenous thermal ablation, the vein was closed through heat induced collagen contraction. However since 2004, we have suggested that although that contraction does occur, transmural heat-induced cell death is essential for fibrosis and atrophy, resulting in effective permanent vein closure and total elimination of venous reflux in the truncal vein[8,9]. With fibrotic occlusion, not only will no blood flow be observed on ultrasound, but one year after surgery the vein itself will have been ingested by the body's immune system and will have disappeared almost entirely.

Using thermal energy to kill the cells of the vein wall in this way is a very effective mechanism, and may account for the high success rate obtained in mid– long term research studies discussed in the literature[10-13]. Therefore, it is not surprising that thermal ablation has been recommended by the National Institute of Health and Care Excellence in the United Kingdom and by the European Society for Vascular Surgery as the most appropriate treatment for truncal venous reflux[14,15].

Endovenous laser ablation (EVLA)

EVLA was first described by Boné in 1999[16], and it can now be used to treat incompetent lower limb truncal veins and perforator veins.

EVLA is a minimally invasive catheter-based device that either emits energy in the visible light range or the microwave range, most commonly at 810 nm and 1470 nm wavelengths, targeting a haemoglobin or water chromophore respectively. Previously, before doctors fully understood how thermal ablation treated truncal venous reflux, endovenous thermal devices were developed that targeted haemoglobin (810 nm). However, if the vein is not fully exsanguinated, and if such a device is used, the blood in the vein lumen may thrombose. Conversely, as the vein wall is white and there is no red pigment or haemoglobin in the vein wall, if the vein is fully exsanguinated then transmural vein wall cell death may not occur completely. Either of these situations can result in thrombotic occlusion with living cells in the surrounding vein wall. We know from previous research that after stripping, a haematoma and living endothelium are the requirements for neovascularisation[17]. In thrombotic occlusion, the vein may appear to be closed on ultrasound for many months or even years, as the lumen is filled with a blood clot. However, over time the vein may re-canalise and hence "re-open", causing recurrent reflux and recurrent varicose veins.

Laser energy from EVLA catheters can be projected straight ahead or to the side, and these different types of laser fibre are appropriately termed forward firing and radial firing fibres respectively. There is some recent research suggesting advantages of the radial firing laser fibres. This is understandable as radial fibres project energy directly into the target vein wall. This early research has shown a more homogenous and effective thermal distribution from these laser fibres relative to forward firing laser fibres[18].

When using a forward firing laser fibre, it is important to remember that this energy is projected straight ahead through the vein lumen and not directly into the target that you want to hit (the vein wall). As such, problems may arise, especially when ablating a truncal vein near the junction with the deep vein. For a forward firing laser fibre, when thermal ablation of the Great Saphenous Vein (GSV) is started too close to the saphenofemoral junction (SFJ), a thrombus may be formed that extends into, or develops within, the common femoral vein, causing an endovenous heat induced thrombosis (EHIT) or a deep vein thrombosis (DVT) respectively[19,20]. Hence, it is recommended to place the laser tip at a distance of approximately 2 cm distal from the SFJ[19].

However, patients vary in anatomy, and in particular, in the size of the GSV to be treated. Therefore, rather than using standard pull-back measurements to treat all GSVs in the same way, we have designed the bubble trap technique that allows doctors to tailor endovenous laser treatment with a forward firing laser device to every patient, while minimising any adverse risk.

The Bubble trap technique

When treating the GSV using a 1470 nm jacket tipped forward firing laser fibre, the vein is percutaneously accessed distally, just below the knee, and the fibre is advanced proximally towards the SFJ under ultrasound control.

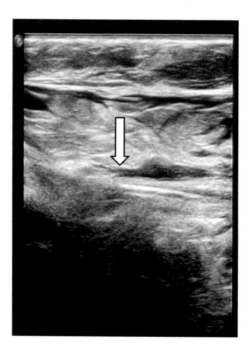

Figure 1: B-Mode (greyscale) ultrasound showing a jacket tipped forward firing endovenous laser fibre (white arrow) within the GSV, just distal to the junction with the epigastric vein

In the bubble trap technique, we initially place the tip of the laser fibre immediately distal to the junction with the inferior epigastric vein (see Figure 1). This will be repositioned later before treatment commences as below. The patient is placed 30 degrees head down to empty the vein. Tumescent anaesthesia is then injected around the GSV.

Upon activation of the laser, any water in the immediate area will be heated and steam bubbles will be generated, which dilate the vein and push the vein wall (the target) away from the laser energy (Figure 2). Therefore compression is applied externally by the ultrasound transducer held longitudinally at the level of the laser tip, to compress the SFJ, pushing the target (vein wall) into

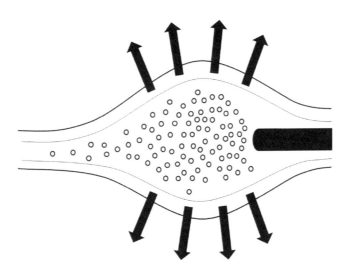

Figure 2: Diagram representing the dilation of the vein wall when a forward firing endovenous laser is activated, due to steam bubble formation and expansion.

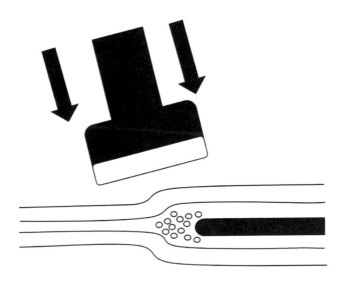

Figure 3: Diagram showing how external pressure from an ultrasound transducer pushes the vein wall (target) into the laser energy, and traps the bubbles. These can be observed on ultrasound ensuring thermal energy is kept within the GSV and does not escape into the deep vein.

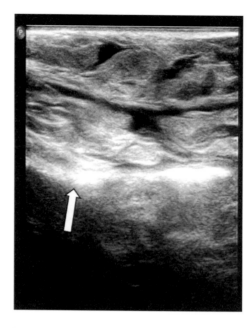

Figure 4: Same patient as in figure 1 when the endovenous laser is activated briefly. Bubbles are seen (white arrow) streaming into the deep vein through the SFJ, potentially damaging the wall of the deep vein, increasing the risk of endothelial damage and thrombosis.

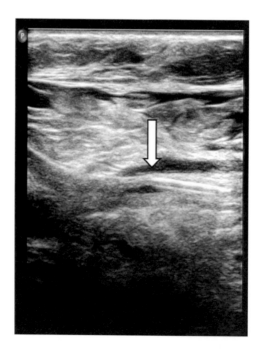

Figure 5: the same patient as figure 1 and 4, where the laser tip is withdrawn 2 to 3 mm (white arrow).

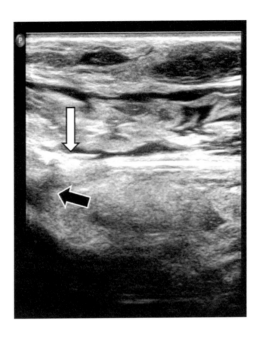

Figure 6: Same patient as figure 1, 4 and 5. The bubbles are trapped in the proximal GSV (white arrow), with no bubbles – and hence no destructive thermal energy – moving into the deep veins through the SFJ (black arrow).

the ablative energy, and to "trap" the bubbles within the GSV. The bubbles are visualised under ultrasound, and used as a marker of thermal energy in our Bubble Trap technique. This uses external compression together with tumescent anaesthesia to allow ablation of the proximal GSV without energy spreading into the deep vein (Figure 3).

Placement of the laser fibre proceeds under ultrasound-guidance. For most cases, the tip is placed about 5 mm distal to the junction of the inferior epigastric vein and the GSV. If the GSV is very dilated, then the tip may be placed further away. When the doctor thinks that the tip is in the correct place, the laser is activated very briefly (<0.25 sec). If bubbles formed at the tip stream proximally through the SFJ and into the Common Femoral Vein the fibre is too close (Figure 4). If this happens, the wall of the deep veins may be damaged by this heat, increasing the risk of endothelial damage and thrombosis. The fibre is withdrawn 2-3 mm (Figure 5), and the process is repeated until the bubbles remain trapped within the GSV (Figure 6). This ensures that there is no spread of destructive thermal energy through the SFJ and into the Common Femoral Vein. Knowing that heat energy is confined to the GSV, normal ablation is commenced. Compression is maintained at the groin for the first 5 cm of laser withdrawal to ensure there is no possibility of proximal streaming of the laser energy via steam bubbles into the deep veins.

Discussion

Compressing the proximal GSV in this way stops vein dilation due to steam formation, and pushes the vein wall (the target for thermal ablation) in front of the laser tip and into the ablative energy stream. With this technique, the heat energy is restricted to the area around the tip of the laser fibre, evidenced by confinement of steam bubbles within the GSV. The bubble trap technique overcomes all problems; it prevents proximal thermal streaming through the SFJ, enabling safe proximal GSV ablation, and is sufficiently flexible to be tailored to each individual GSV.

Compression of the SFJ has been recommended by the Australian College of Phlebology clinical procedure guidelines for EVLA[21]. This document acknowledges sufficient placement of tumescent anaesthesia around the proximal vein section and external compression using the ultrasound probe to protect the femoral vein from thermal energy, while still maintaining a laser fibre distance of 1 to 3 cm from the junction. Our technique is unique as it combines proximal compression, with accurate visualisation of the bubbles produced upon laser activation. There are two reasons why the "bubble trap" component to this technique is so important; firstly, to ensure safe proximal ablation with accurate ultrasound visualisation and secondly, to close the vein as flush as possible to the junction of the inferior epigastric vein and the GSV, reducing any blind "sinus" of GSV in which thrombus might form.

We have been using and teaching this technique since 2013 when we first started using the forward firing laser fibre. We have had no incidence of DVT, EHIT or proximal recanalization while using this technique, in over 921 cases. Furthermore, no patient has returned with recurrence from another tributary of the SFJ, once thought to be a reason to perform a flush ligation.

It is important to acknowledge that our incidence of DVT and EHIT are significantly lower than the reported figures in clinical audits from other units reported across the literature. This may be due to the pullback being started without adequate compression or accurate visualisation of thermal energy spread in real time during the procedure. One study has reported reduced incidence of EHIT with a laser pullback starting 2.5 cm back from the SFJ compared to that of 2 cm[19]. The authors therefore concluded that initiating ablation further back from the SFJ is safer. However, this reduced incidence may be the result of reduced proximal thermal streaming of steam bubbles into the deep vein because of the added distance. More likely though, it is due to an increased chance of a patent tributary joining the longer section of untreated GSV stump, 'washing out' the section of vein, preventing the risk of thrombus formation.

Therefore, by recommending to pull the laser fibre back approximately 2 cm from the SFJ, without also ensuring proximal compression and visualisation of heat distribution using ultrasound, thrombotic occlusion may develop in the vein region immediately proximal to the tip of the laser fibre, resulting in EHIT or even DVT by thrombus extension. Despite the laser fibre placement guideline of 2cm being widely recommended as a safety measure, we suggest that it may enhance the risk of proximal thrombosis with possible deep vein implications, as well as causing inadequate closure of the proximal GSV. We believe that when using forwards firing laser fibres with wavelengths that use water as a chromophore, this region should be treated using the bubble trap technique, which we have demonstrated through experience to be safe and effective.

In 2004, the authors published a case from 1999 of a thrombus formation in the blind end of an ablated GSV, which projected into the common femoral vein[9]. At this stage, it was a novel finding, so the authors took the patient to the operating theatre and excised this thrombus and the proximal GSV. Subsequently in 2005, this sort of thrombus was named EHIT[22]. At open removal of this thrombus, it was clear that the body of the thrombus had formed in the proximal part of the GSV that was still patent. The body of the thrombus did not extend beyond this part, and only a thin tail of thrombus extended into the common femoral vein through the SFJ. This was clearly due to the inferior epigastric vein allowing flow through this proximal part of the GSV and SFJ, preventing occlusive thrombus forming here. From Virchow's triad and experience of veins, it is clear that a thrombus can form where there is a blind ending sac within the venous system. As such, it is the aim of any ablation technique to close a vein as flush as possible to a tributary orifice. In the proximal GSV, the most easily observed tributary is the inferior epigastric vein. In addition, this vein drains the lower abdominal wall and when left untreated, does not contribute towards the development of leg varicose veins. Hence, it is logical to try and close the GSV flush with the junction between this vein and the SFJ. This is exactly what the bubble trap technique achieves.

The often quoted "2 cm back from the SFJ" guideline appears to have arisen as an arbitrary "safety" measure, with no preceding evidence to verify this measurement. The fact that this is illogical as a cast-iron rule is proven by the Transluminal Occlusion of Perforator (TRLOP) procedure that is used for the closure of incompetent perforating veins where a gap of 2 cm from the junction with the deep vein would mean the fibre would often be outside of the leg! Also, a 5-year review of TRLOP highlighted only one incidence of DVT[23].

In conclusion, positioning the fibre 2 cm from the SFJ appears to be an unsupported dogma. We present a new technique utilising ultrasound visualisation and compression that allows the GSV to be closed proximally from the junction with the inferior epigastric vein using EVLA with a forward firing laser and water specific wavelengths. This technique allows safe and effective ablation of the proximal GSV, and each ablation case to be modified and tailored for every patient.

References

1. Munasinghe A, Smith C, Kianifard B, Price BA, Holdstock JM, Whiteley MS. Strip-track revascularisation after stripping of the great saphenous vein. Br J Surg. 2007; 94 (7): 840-3.

2. Ostler AE, Holdstock JM, Harrison CC, Price BA, Whiteley MS. Strip-tract revascularization as a source of recurrent venous reflux following high saphenous tie and stripping: results at 5–8 years after surgery. Phlebology. 2015; 30 (8): 569-72.

3. Jones L, Braithwaite BD, Selwyn D, Cooke S, Earnshaw JJ. Neovascularisation is the principal cause of varicose vein recurrence: results of a randomised trial of stripping the long saphenous vein. Eur J Vasc Endovasc Surg. 1996; 12: 442–445.

4. ElKaffas H, ElKashef O, ElBaz W. Great saphenous vein radiofrequency ablation versus standard stripping in the management of primary varicose veins- a randomized clinical trial. Angiology. 2001; 62 (1): 49-54.

5. Lurie F, Creton D, Eklof B, Kabnick LS Kirstner RL, Pichot O et al. Prospective randomized

study of endovenous radiofrequency obliteration (closure procedure) versus ligation and stripping in a selected patient population (EVOLVeS Study). J Vasc Surg. 2003; 38 (2): 207-14.

6.   Rasmussen LH, Lawaetz M, Bjoern L, Vennits B, Blemings A, Eklof B. Randomized clinical trial comparing endovenous laser ablation, radiofrequency ablation, foam sclerotherapy and surgical stripping for great saphenous varicose veins. Br J Surg. 2011; 98 (8): 1079-87.

7.   Kianifard B, Holdstock JM, Whiteley MS. Radiofrequency ablation (VNUS closure) does not cause neo-vascularisation at the groin at one year: results of a case controlled study. Surgeon. 2006; 4 (2): 71-4.

8.   Mark Whiteley. New Methods of Vein Ablation. In: Venous Disease Simplified Eds: Alun H Davies, Tim Lees & Ian F Lane. UK: Harley 2006.

9.   Whiteley MS, Holdstock JM. Percutaneous radiofrequency ablations of Varicose Veins (VNUS Closure). In: Vascular and Endovascular Challenges. Roger M Greenhalgh, editor. London; BIBA Publishing 2004. p 361- 381.

10.   Fassiadis N, Kianifard B, Holdstock JM, Whiteley MS. Ultrasound changes at the saphenofemoral junction and in the long saphenous vein during the first year of VNUS Closure. Int Angiol. 2002; 21 (3): 272-4.

11.   Taylor DC, Whiteley AM, Fernandez-Hart TJ, Whiteley MS. Ten year results of radiofrequency ablation (VNUS Closure®) of the great saphenous and anterior accessory saphenous veins, in the treatment of varicose veins. Phlebology. 2013; 28 (6): 335.

12.   Nicolini P, The Closure Group. Treatment of primary varicose veins by endovenous obliteration with the VNUS closure system: results of a prospective multicentre study. Eur J Vasc Endovasc Surg. 2005; 29 (4): 433-9.

13.   Merchant RF, Pichot O, The Closure Study Group. Long-term outcomes of endovenous radiofrequency obliteration of saphenous reflux as a treatment for superficial venous insufficiency. J Vasc Surg. 2005; 42 (3): 502-9.

14.   NICE (National Institute for Health and Care Excellence) clinical guidelines - CG 168. Varicose veins in the legs: the diagnosis and management of varicose veins. Issued July 2013.

15.   Wittens C, Davies AH, Baekgaard N et al. Editors Choice – Management of Chronic Venous Disease: practive guidelines of the European society for vascular surgery. Eur J Vasc Endovasc Surg. 2015; 49: 678-737.

16.   Boné C. Tratamiento endoluminal de las varices con laser de diodo: estudio preliminary. Rev Patol Vasc. 1999; 5: 35– 46.

17.   Ostler AE, Holdstock JM, Harrison CC, Price BA, Whiteley MS. Strip-tract revascularization as a source of recurrent venous reflux following high saphenous tie and stripping: results at 5–8 years after surgery. Phlebology. 2015; 30 (8): 569-72.

18.   Ashpitel H, Salguero F, La Ragione R, Whiteley M. Radial-firing endovenous laser penetrates deeper into the vein wall than forward-firing jacket-tipped fibers and reduces carbonization – an *ex vivo* study using histology and immunohistochemistry. J Vasc Surg Venous lymphat

disord. 2017; 5(1): 147-8.

19. Sadek M, Kabnick LS, Rockman CB, Berland TL, Zhou D, Chasin C, Jacobowitz GR, Adelman MA. Increasing ablation distance peripheral to the saphenofemoral junction may result in a diminished rate of endothermal heat-induced thrombosis. J Vasc Surg Venous Lymphatic Disord. 2013; 1(3): 251-262.

20. Marsh P, Price BA, Holdstock J, Harrison C, Whiteley MS. Deep vein thrombosis (DVT) after thermoablation techniques: rates of endovenous heat-induced thrombosis (EHIT) and classical DVT after radiofrequency and endovenous laser ablation in a single center. Eur J Vasc Endovasc sur. 2010; 40(4): 521-527

21. Australasian College of Phlebology. Endovenous Laser Ablation Clinical Procedures Standard. Appendix 1 to endovenous laser ablation standard. 2010. http://www.phlebology.com.au/standards

22. Kabnick LS, Ombrellino M, Agis H, Mortiz M, Almeida J, Baccaglini U, et al. Endovenous heat induced thrombus (EHIT) at the superficial- deep venous junction: a new post-treatment clinical entity, clas- sification and potential treatment strategies. 18th Annual Meeting of the American Venous Forum, Miami, Florida; 2006.

23. Bacon JL, Dinneen AJ, Marsh P, Holdstock JM, Price BA, Whiteley MS. Five-year results of incompetent perforator vein closure using TRans-luminal Occlusion of Perforator. Phlebology.2009; 24(2): 74-78.

Chapter 8

Radial Endovenous Laser

Author
James Lawson

Institution
Skin and Vein clinic Oosterwal Alkmaar, Department of vascular surgery

Introduction

For several decades high ligation at the saphenofemoral junction and stripping of the GSV (HL/S) was the treatment of choice in order to eradicate saphenous vein reflux. Endovenous laser ablation (EVLA) was introduced around the turn of the millennium as an alternative to open ligation and stripping of incompetent saphenous veins. The electromagnetic energy from near infrared light was brought intraluminal via a bare glass fibre. Laser energy is absorbed by blood or vein wall and transformed into heat energy damaging the vein wall by cell destruction and collagen denaturation causing occlusion. In many publications it was concluded that this less invasive treatment modality reduced postoperative pain, morbidity and cost with acceptable short- and long-term results. Mostly a comparison was made with open surgery under general or spinal anaesthesia without duplex guidance[1].

Like Rasmussen, we published a randomized trial (2010) in which we compared high ligation and stripping with bare tip EVLA 980 nm using both tumescent anaesthesia and duplex guidance. There was no statistically significant difference in efficacy between EVLA and stripping in both studies but it showed that from the 4th postoperative day EVLA patients had more postoperative pain than open surgery[2,3]. So when stripping is performed using ultrasound-guided tumescent anaesthesia the recovery profile is more or less similar to bare tip EVLA. A bare cutting fibre tends to perforate the venous wall causing postoperative pain and haematoma. White blood cell extravasation causes inflammation after a few days inducing pain as well. Bare tip fibres mostly cause only local injury at one site of the vein wall.

Rather than inducing a completely circular thermal damage of the vein wall it leaves only small, locally damaged wall areas, which can lead to a higher frequency of non-occlusion. Circular damage is needed to prevent recanalization. A higher wavelength and modification of the laser tip is suggested in order to avoid these kind of complications[4].

Is there another recovery profile with the use of different wavelengths?

There are different theories about the thermal effect on the vein wall during EVLA: direct absorption of the laser light, indirect heating of the vein wall by endovenous steam bubble formation and direct damage of the vein wall by direct contact with the laser fibre tip causing carbonization.

Collagen denaturation and constriction will eventually close the vein permanently[5]. Laser light is monochromatic and by definition has a narrow bandwidth so it can target chromophores selectively. The chromophores for the lower wavelengths are haemoglobin or myoglobin, whereas with the higher wavelengths the chromophore is water, with the laser energy exciting the water molecules to a state of higher energy. Energy release to surrounding tissue damages the tissue by heat through photochemical and photothermolytic mechanisms[6].

The optical chromophore of the vein wall is water so the use of higher wavelength should be a more effective and efficient option. As the wavelength of light increases so does the depth of penetration into the tissue. 1470 nm lasers have higher absorption in water, theoretically 40 times more than with 810, 940 or 980 nm lasers[7]. According to the mathematical modelling by Mordon[8] the optical excitation is much higher at 1470 nm (4 to 9 times higher) than with the shorter wavelengths, allowing the use of less power for the same efficiency. The problem is that there is always a lot of scattering of light in tissue usually reducing the penetration into the target tissue. Broadening the incident beam occurs, decreasing the effective fluence in the target area[9]. However, heat is also transmitted by conduction to the tissue surrounding the target area. *In vitro* experiments in blood and water showed that 1470nm has a higher absorption in blood and water, with lower power settings and so if you want to focus on the vein wall during treatment, a bloodless vein is preferable. This can be supported by tumescent compression and the leg in a Trendelenburg position.

A major side effect of endovenous laser ablation is postoperative pain and bruising. A few studies have reported that patients treated with higher wavelength lasers had lower postoperative pain scores, used lower amounts of pain-killers and developed less haematoma[10,11]. Others found no difference between the use of different wavelengths and adverse events[12,13].

In conclusion, the evidence to support the efficiency and beneficial effect on the postoperative course of higher-wavelength vs lower-wavelength laser fibres remains controversial. There seems no difference in effectiveness in terms of recanalization or recurrence of disease.

Modification of the fibre tip

To avoid vein wall perforations caused by a hot bare tip of the laser fibre, several improvements have been suggested and investigated. The jacket-tip fibre called "NeverTouch" (AngioDynamics, Inc., Queensbury, NY) is a glass fibre where the distal tip of the fibre is protected by a jacket that is covering the hot portion of the fibre from the vein wall during treatment. Besides protection of the vein wall the jacket has also a glass weld at the distal tip of a 600 μm fibre. This weld results in an effective fibre diameter of 905 μm and lowers the actual power density by 56% from that of a standard bare-tip 600 μm fibre. The net effect is a homogeneous ablation with less focal charring of the vein wall than that which is seen with bare-tip fibres. Small size comparative studies with bare-tip fibres show better postoperative recovery and less pain if jacket-tip fibres are used[14,15].

A retrospective comparative study showed a five-fold increase in the recanalisation rate for veins treated with EVLA using the NeverTouch gold-tip fibre compared with standard bare-tip fibres[16].

With the same philosophy a tulip fibre has been developed. The use of a tulip fibre avoids this direct contact since the fibre tip is centred intra-luminally. This results in a more homogenous energy distribution to the vein wall. A randomized study comparing tulip fibre and bare-tip fibre showed equal occlusion rates with a better recovery profile and postoperative quality of life in patients treated with the tulip fibre[17,18].

In both treatments however, carbonization could affect the distal part of the tip which, as a consequence, could result in a reduction of beam diffusion and high temperatures damaging the distal tip.

The reason to develop laser fibres with a radial laser light emission was to produce a circular radiation of the light directly to the vein wall. There is a direct heating of tissue rather than first heating of the surrounding blood with subsequent conduction of heat to the vein wall by steam bubbles[19]. Sroka (2013) revealed in *ex vivo* experiments with a cow's foot that with the radial fibre the fluence rate is significantly reduced below the ablation threshold[20]. It results in a circumferential applied irradiation with a fluence rate of 75 W/cm^2 in comparison with 525 W/cm^2 from a bare tip fibre which is above the ablation threshold under the same circumstances. The circular damage takes place in a circumferential homogenous manner. As in radiofrequency ablation there is a denaturation and contraction of collagen fibres which guarantees a complete and durable occlusion after fibrosis of the vein. With a blunt fibre tip and diffusion of the laser light with lower power density, perforation of the vein wall will not normally occur. Carbonization of the tip that usually occurs during thermal ablation with the use of bare fibre is almost non-existent with radial fibres. Shrinkage occurs immediately during treatment which gives a sticky and pulling sensation on the fibre during pull back.

Spreafico[21] compared the histology of the treated vein after using a 980 nm and 1470 nm bare tip fibre with the 1470 nm radial fibre. The 980 nm and 1470 nm bare tip fibres only caused damage to the vein wall in the areas of contact, resulting in charring, vaporization and inhomogeneous ablation with varied depth and perforations. Radial fibres did not show any contact damage with the intima, but instead showed a deep coagulative necrosis of the intima and media, together with vacuolizations and fissures in the sub-intimal area.

Pannier (2011) performed a 6 months prospective study on 50 patients after endovenous GSV ablation with a radial fibre using cold tumescent anaesthesia. During the same session all insufficient tributaries were treated by phlebectomy. Postoperative recovery was smooth with Visual Analogue Scores (VAS) for pain below 1, during the first 2 weeks (Scale 1-5). Furthermore, 80 % of patients didn't have any signs of ecchymosis. Return to daily activities was possible after an average of 1.6 days (SD 1.1)[4]. Occlusion rate was 100 % after 6 months.

The linear endovenous energy density (LEED, J/cm), which was thought necessary for the occlusion of the vein, was calculated by the following formula: 10 × vein diameter (D, mm) in the upright position. The average LEED was 90.8 J/cm vein with a minimum of 46.2 J/cm and a maximum of 188.5 J/cm (SD 35.3). The only complications were found in 3 patients (6%) who were suffering from a permanent paraesthesia. The high rate of this nerve damage was probably caused by the high LEED during treatment[22].

Schwarz (2010)[23] conducted a prospective, non-randomized observational cohort study of 312 consecutively treated GSV's in 286 patients. Of these, a bare laser fibre (ELVeS-plus kit) was used to treat 168 legs in 150 patients and a radial fibre (ELVeS-radial kit) was used in 144 legs in 136 patients. Ecchymosis and bruising were significantly less frequent after treatment with the radial fibre than after the bare fibre (P < 0.0001). No DVT occurred after radial fibre treatment. The occlusion rate was 100 % after 3 months.

In a prospective randomized study of 60 patients, Doganci found that side effects such as pain, induration, ecchymosis and paraesthesia were significantly reduced with the 1470 nm laser and radial fibre system compared to the 980 nm bare-tip laser fibre[24]. The paraesthesia rate was 10 % (3/30) vs 30 % (9/30) after the bare fibre. Return to daily activities was faster after ablation using the radial fibre (1.6 v 2.3 days). The 6 month closure was 100% after both treatments.

In 2010, we performed a postoperative recovery study to compare High Saphenous Ligation and Stripping (HL/S) with endovenous laser ablation using (EVLA) a bare tip fibre with a 980 nm laser, a radial fibre using a 1470 nm laser (Biolitec) and segmental "radiofrequency" ablation with VNUS Closure FAST[25]. All procedures were performed under local tumescent anaesthesia and were well

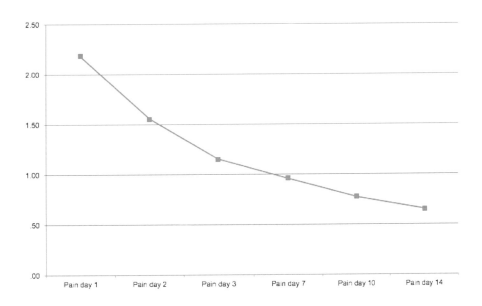

Figure 1: Mean VAS pain scores after EVLA with radial fibre

tolerated.

Postoperative pain was significantly less after the VNUS Closure FAST procedure compared with the other treatments. The intensity of postoperative pain was significant and most explicit in the second week after the EVLA 980 nm procedure. Quality of Life (QoL) results were most favourable in the VNUS Closure FAST group. After both VNUS Closure FAST and EVLA with ELVeS Radial 1470 nm, patients resumed daily activities after +/-1.4 days (mean). After HL/S and EVLA with ELVeS 980 nm, the interval was +/-3.2 days (mean). Return to work was significantly faster after VNUS Closure FAST and EVLA with ELVeS Radial 1470 nm (mean +/- 2.9 days) compared with +/- 4.2 days after HL/S and EVLA with ELVeS 980nm.

In our ongoing randomized study comparing VNUS Closure FAST against radial fibre with 1470 nm laser, 140 patients (174 legs) treated with radial fibre thermal ablation of the GSV were followed for a maximum of 24 months. After 12 months, 138 legs were seen and after 24 months, 68 legs were reviewed. The average linear endovenous energy density (LEED) was 77.8 J/cm vein (SD 10.4), post-operative VAS pain scores were low (mean <1; see Fig 1). Seventy-four percent of patients did not use pain medication at all. Bruising was seen in fewer than 19 % of treated legs. Carbonization of the tip was not observed. Time to resume normal activities was a mean of 1.13 days. The mean time to return to work was 2.17 days (SD 2.26). Small areas of hypoaesthesia in the lower leg were still present after 1 year in 2.9 % (4/138). Endovenous Heat Induced Thrombus (EHIT) Class 2 was detected after 2 procedures with spontaneous resolution. A thrombotic complication was seen in 1 leg (crural vein occlusion). Great saphenous vein occlusion rate (measured 3 cm distal from the junction) after 12 months was 98.5 % (136/138) and after 24 months was 97.2 % (66/68). There was a significant improvement from the AVVQ and VCSS one and two years after surgery.

Discussion

Measuring, reporting and comparing outcomes are important steps toward rapidly improving patient results and making good choices about reducing costs[26]. Costs are not only the real costs of the procedure but the immediate and persistent health gain saving costs for society in terms of preventing absence from work. So outcomes should include the health gain most relevant to patients and society. That means short-term safety, fast recovery and long-term functionality in terms of quality of life. Porter (2010) arrayed health outcome in a three-tiered hierarchy:

- Tier 1 is improvement of health.
- Tier 2 is the disutility of the care process.
- Tier 3 is the long term benefit of the treatment.

The effects of treatment should be sustainable without recurrence and new health problems as a consequence of the treatment (long term complications). The best treatment has the fastest recovery and fastest time to return to normal activities and work, with the same or better health improvement in both the short and long term as other alternatives. That means avoiding diagnostic errors, ineffective care, treatment-related discomfort, complications and adverse effects.

Some systematic reviews favoured thermal ablation above open surgery like High Ligation and

Stripping (HL/S)[1,27] in treating saphenous reflux. Results could be biased because of pooling effects of observational studies with some mix of randomized trials[28]. Siribumrungwong (2012)[28] conducted a very well designed and statistically sound meta-analysis of only RCTs comparing all relevant outcomes in all tiers including efficacies (i.e. primary failure and clinical recurrence), postoperative complications (i.e. wound infection, paraesthesia, superficial thrombophlebitis, haematoma and ecchymosis), postoperative pain, time to return to normal activities or work and QOL between these endovenous ablations and surgery, and also between themselves.

A composite outcome of clinical recurrence (primary failure, reflux in tributaries and neovascularisation) showed no difference between endovenous and open surgery. QOL at a later stage in the EVLA and surgery groups were not significantly different. Pain scores after treatment were significantly lower after radiofrequency ablation (RFA) but not after EVLA in comparison with open surgery. In 4 RCT's postoperative pain was higher after EVLA v Surgery[2,3,29,30]. In 2 RCT's no difference was found[31,32].

Return to normal activities or work was significantly shorter for RFA but not for EVLA compared with surgery. It must be mentioned that all studies were performed with 810 and 980 nm bare tip fibres. Return to normal activities and work following open varicose vein surgery, is highly variable and independent of doctor's advice[33]. The median back to work was 14 days (7-21). In our study there was no difference between EVLA 980 nm and HL/S (4.38 v 4.15 days)3. Both procedures were performed under tumescent anaesthesia. In Rasmussens study[34] both procedures were done under tumescent anaesthesia, with no difference in time to return to work (7.0 v 7.6 days). In RCT's where open surgery was performed under general anaesthesia and EVLA under tumescence, return to normal activities and work is also dependent on the type of anaesthesia and comparisons under such circumstances are not always valuable.

In order to improve the postoperative recovery with less postoperative pain after EVLA in comparison to open surgery, a modification of the way of emitting the laser light from the fibre along with using a higher wavelength is likely to be a solution to avoid perforations and other complications found with a bare tip fibre. Our own experience, and that of other different authors, has shown that the radial fibre gives a homogeneous energy deposition to the vein wall with lower power density and without axial irradiance transmission. Together with the empty vein technique (Trendelenburg position of the patient and a larger volume of tumescent fluid) the postoperative period is usually uneventful without vein perforations and with minimal post-operative pain and bruising/haematoma in most patients. Normal activities can start immediately. We advise the patient to go back to work the same or next day after EVLA with a radial fibre as we do with patients following an RFA treatment. High occlusion rates after a follow up of 2 years gives us confidence that the efficacy of the radial fiber is at least equal to bare-tip lasers

References

1. Van den Bos R, Arends L, Kockaert M, Neumann M, Nijsten T. Endovenous therapies of lower extremity varicosities: A meta-analysis. J Vasc Surg. 2009;49(1):230–9.

2. Rasmussen LH, Lawaetz M, Bjoern L, Vennits B, Blemings A, Eklof B. Randomized clinical trial comparing endovenous laser ablation, radiofrequency ablation, foam sclerotherapy and surgical stripping for great saphenous varicose veins. Br J Surg. 2011;98(8):1079–87.

3. Pronk P, Gauw SA, Mooij MC, Gaastra MTW, Lawson JA, van Goethem AR, et al. Randomised controlled trial comparing sapheno-femoral ligation and stripping of the great saphenous vein with endovenous laser ablation (980 nm) using local tumescent anaesthesia: one year results. Eur J Vasc Endovasc Surg. 2010 ;40(5):649–56.

4. Pannier F, Rabe E, Rits J, Kadiss A, Maurins U. Endovenous laser ablation of great saphenous veins using a 1470 nm diode laser and the radial fibre - follow-up after six months. Phlebology / Venous Forum of the Royal Society of Medicine. 2011;26(1):35–9.

5. Massaki ABMN, Kiripolsky MG, Detwiler SP, Goldman MP. Endoluminal laser delivery mode and wavelength effects on varicose veins in an *Ex vivo* model. Weiss RA, Geronemus RG, editors. Lasers Surg. Med. 2013;45(2):123–9.

6. De Felice E. Shedding light: laser physics and mechanism of action. Phlebology. 2010;25(1):11–28.

7. Almeida J, Mackay E, Javier J, Mauriello J, Raines J. Saphenous laser ablation at 1470 nm targets the vein wall, not blood. Vascular and endovascular surgery. 2009;43(5):467–72.

8. Mordon SR, Wassmer B, Zemmouri J. Mathematical modeling of 980-nm and 1320-nm endovenous laser treatment. Lasers Surg. Med. 2007;39(3):256–65.

9. Vuylsteke ME, Mordon SR. Endovenous Laser Ablation: A Review of Mechanisms of Action. Annals of vascular surgery. Annals of Vascular Surgery Inc. 2012;26(3):424–33.

10. Proebstle TM, Moehler T, Gül D, Herdemann S. Endovenous treatment of the great saphenous vein using a 1,320 nm Nd:YAG laser causes fewer side effects than using a 940 nm diode laser. Dermatologic surgery. 2005;31(12):1678–83; discussion1683–4.

11. Kabnick LS. Outcome of different endovenous laser wavelengths for great saphenous vein ablation. J Vasc Surg. 2006;43(1):88–93.

12. van den Bos RR, van Ruijven PWM, van der Geld CWM, van Gemert MJC, Neumann HAM, Nijsten T. Endovenous Simulated Laser Experiments at 940 and 1470nm Suggest Wavelength-Independent Temperature Profiles. Eur J Vasc Endovasc Surg. 2012;44(1):77–81.

13. Duman E, Yildirim E, Saba T, Ozulku M, Gunday M, Coban G. The effect of laser wavelength on postoperative pain score in the endovenous ablation of saphenous vein insufficiency. Diagn Interv Radiol. 2013; 19:326–329

14. Kabnick L. Are There Differences Between Bare, Covered, Or Diffusion Fibers For Endovenous Treatment of the Great Saphenous Vein? Proceedings Veith Symposium 2008.

15. Kabnick LSK. Which is More Important for Postoperative Recovery: Laser Wavelength or Fibers? J Vasc Surg. 2012 ;55(1):307.

16. Prince EA, Soares GM, Silva M, Taner A, Ahn S, Dubel GJ, et al. Impact of Laser Fiber Design on Outcome of Endovenous Ablation of Lower-Extremity Varicose Veins: Results

from a Single Practice. Cardiovasc Intervent Radiol. 2010 ;34(3):536–41.

17. Vuylsteke M, Van Dorpe J, Roelens J, De Bo T, Mordon S, Fourneau I. Intraluminal Fibre-Tip Centring can Improve Endovenous Laser Ablation: A Histological Study. Eur J Vasc Endovasc Surg. 2010 40(1):110–6.

18. Vuylsteke ME, Thomis S, Mahieu P, Mordon S, Fourneau I. Endovenous Laser Ablation of the Great Saphenous Vein Using a Bare Fibre versus a Tulip Fibre: A Randomised Clinical Trial. Eur J Vasc Endovasc Surg. 2012 :1–6.

19. Sroka R, Weick K, Sadeghi-Azandaryani M, Steckmeier B, Schmedt C-G. Endovenous laser therapy - application studies and latest investigations. J Biophoton. 2010 ;3(5-6):269–76.

20. Sroka R, Pongratz T, Siegrist K, Burgmeier C, Barth HD, Schmedt C-G. Endovenous Laser Application. Phlebologie. 2013;42(3):121–9.

21. Spreafico G, Giardino R, MD AP, Iaderosa G, Pavei P, Giraldi E, et al. Histological damage of saphenous venous wall treated *in vivo* with radial fiber and 1470 nm diode laser. J Vasc Endovasc Surg. 2011;18:1-2

22. Arnez A, Kiser R, Lakhanpal S, Nguyen K. Letter regarding: F Pannier, E Rabe, J Rits, A Kadiss, U Maurins. Endovenous laser ablation of great saphenous veins using a 1470 nm diode laser and the radial fibre - follow-up after six months. Phlebology. 2012;27(2):101–1.

23. Schwarz T, Hodenberg von E, Furtwängler C, Rastan A, Zeller T, Neumann F-J. Endovenous laser ablation of varicose veins with the 1470-nm diode laser. J Vasc Surg. 2010; 51(6):1474–8.

24. Doganci S, Demirkilic U. Comparison of 980 nm laser and bare-tip fibre with 1470 nm laser and radial fibre in the treatment of great saphenous vein varicosities: a prospective randomised clinical trial. Eur J Vasc Endovasc Surg. 2010; 40(2):254–9.

25. P Pronk, S A Gauw, M C Mooij, M T W Gaastra, J A Lawson and C J van Vlijmen-van Keulen A prospective recovery study after high ligation and stripping or endovenous treatment of the insufficient great saphenous vein using local anaesthesia. Phlebology. 2010; 25(6):296–311.

26. Porter ME. What is value in health care? N Engl J Med. 2010; 363(26):2477–81.

27. Luebke T, Gawenda M, Heckenkamp J, Brunkwall J. Meta-analysis of endovenous radiofrequency obliteration of the great saphenous vein in primary varicosis. J Endovasc Ther. 2008 :15(2):213–23.

28. Siribumrungwong B, Noorit P, Wilasrusmee C, Attia J, Thakkinstian A. A Systematic Review and Meta-analysis of Randomised Controlled Trials Comparing Endovenous Ablation and Surgical Intervention in Patients with Varicose Vein. Eur J Vasc Endovasc Surg; 2012; 14 :1–10.

29. Rass K, Frings N, Glowacki P, Hamsch C, Graber S, Vogt T, et al. Comparable Effectiveness of Endovenous Laser Ablation and High Ligation With Stripping of the Great Saphenous Vein: Two-Year Results of a Randomized Clinical Trial (RELACS Study).; Arch Dermatol. 2011; 148(1): 49-48.

30. Flessenkämper I, Hartmann M, Stenger D, Roll S. Endovenous laser ablation with and without high ligation compared with high ligation and stripping in the treatment of great saphenous varicose veins: initial results of a multicentre randomized controlled trial. Phlebology. 2013; 28: 16-23.

31. Darwood RJ, Theivacumar N, Dellagrammaticas D, Mavor AID, Gough MJ. Randomized clinical trial comparing endovenous laser ablation with surgery for the treatment of primary great saphenous varicose veins. Br J Surg. 2008; 95: 294–301.

32. Christenson JT, Gueddi S, Gemayel G, Bounameaux H. Prospective randomized trial comparing endovenous laser ablation and surgery for treatment of primary great saphenous varicose veins with a 2-year follow-up. J Vasc Surg. 2010; 52 (5): 1234–41.

33. Darwood RJ, Walker N, Bracey M, Cowan AR, Thompson JF, Campbell WB. Return to Work, Driving and Other Activities After Varicose Vein Surgery is Very Variable and is Influenced Little By Advice From Specialists. Eur J Vasc Endovasc Surg. 2009;38(2):213–9.

34. Rasmussen LH, Bjoern L, Lawaetz M, Blemings A, Lawaetz B, Eklof B. Randomized trial comparing endovenous laser ablation of the great saphenous vein with high ligation and stripping in patients with varicose veins: short-term results. J Vasc Surg. 2007;46(2):308–15.

Chapter 9

Ablation of varicose veins by pulsated steam injection

Author
René Milleret

Institution
Clinique Pasteur, Pézenas, France

Introduction

T. Proebstle postulated in 2003[1] that the vein wall heating observed during endovenous laser ablation was mediated by generation of steam bubbles in the blood. Endovenous laser was recognized as the more efficient technique in a meta-analysis[2]. In 2005, a French physician, Dr Henri Mehier, was beginning to treat cancer experimentally by heating them through direct injection of water vapour (= steam) pulses.

We worked together to devise some equipment able to heat the inside of veins through steam pulses emitted directly from the tip of a catheter. After *in vitro* studies and animal experiments this equipment was tested successfully in patients and is now in clinical use in several European countries (Cerma Vein, Archamps– France).

Material

The generator (Figure 1) comprises of a pouch of sterile water which is passed into a piston pump actuated by compressed air at a pressure of 5 bar. There is no contact between water and the compressed air. The pressurized water is forced to the tip of a hand-piece that can be re-sterilised, where it is heated in a micro tube of 0.1 mm internal diameter. Pulses of steam are emitted with a temperature of 150 °C. A catheter is connected to the hand-piece to transmit the steam into the vein to be treated. Depending on the length of the catheter, the temperature of steam goes down to 120 °C through heat losses along the tubing. Each pulse vaporizes only 0.8 microlitres of water and so there is no haemolysis observed as the total quantity of water injected into the veins is less than 5 ml. Each pulse condensates and relaxes 60 Joules of thermal energy to the tissues.

A single use catheter is used to drive steam into the vein.

2 types of treatment catheter are available (Figure 2):

- Flexi-Vein® is a 60 cm long, 1.2 mm (5F) stainless style straight catheter with Teflon® covering.

It has 2 lateral holes 5 mm from the tip which emit steam without heating the deep veins when close to the junctions.

• Trib-Vein® is shorter at 10 cm long, 0.8 mm (3F) PEEK catheter designed for treating tributaries. It has a hole at the tip, allowing steam under pressure to reach through the bends of tortuous veins.

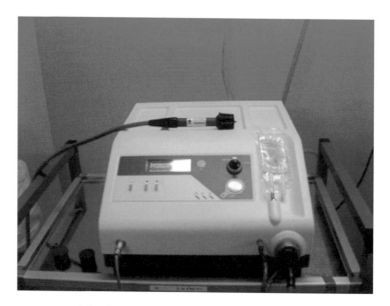

Figure 1: Steam generator with hand piece

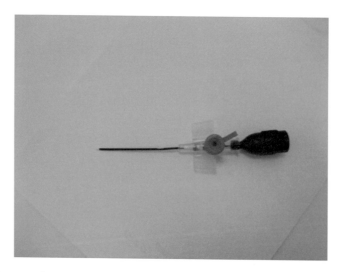

Figure 2: The tributary catheter

Preliminary Studies
In Vitro experiments
Freshly stripped segments of Great Saphenous Vein were treated *in vitro* by the application of repeated pulses of steam. We observed that there was initially a retraction of the vein wall followed by a shortening of the whole segment if heating was continued. The vein wall thickened considerably and was comparable to what is reported after radio-frequency heating. We used these *in vitro* observations to define the optimal parameters to test in the animal studies.

Animal studies
We treated the Small Saphenous Vein (SSV) in the posterior limb of 12 female sheep. Two limbs were heated by segmental radio-frequency ablation (VNUS Venefit® catheter) for comparison purposes. We measured the blood temperature in the Vena Cava and the temperature in the tissues around the treated vein. We also monitored the main pulmonary and circulatory parameters to detect any change that might be induced by the procedure. No general or local adverse effects were observed. Blood temperature in the Vena Cava remained normal. The temperature in the peri-venous tissue went up to 45 °C without tumescence and only up to 37 °C with tumescence fluid injection. Acute (8 days) and chronic (6 months) microscopic studies were performed on the treated veins. All were obliterated at the time of study, with retraction of at least 50 % of the initial calibre. We did not find any damage to peri-venous tissue.

Methods
Treating Saphenous trunks
The procedure is similar to other endovenous thermal ablation techniques. The vein is cannulated with a 16 G Grey infusion catheter (VenFlon®), under ultrasound guidance. The initial puncture point is usually at the upper third of the calf for Great Saphenous Vein and at mid-calf for the Small Saphenous Vein. Catheterization is usually straightforward because the stainless steel Flexi-Vein® catheter acts as a guide wire. If a blockage cannot be crossed by gentle hand manoeuvers a second puncture just above the area of obstruction is advised.

The tip of the catheter is very echogenic, being made of metal. It is positioned 2 cm distal to the sapheno-femoral junction (SFJ) for treatment of the Great Saphenous Vein (GSV) and 3 cm distal to the sapheno-popliteal junction (SPJ) for treatment of the SSV. Tumescent anaesthesia is applied around the vein under ultrasound control. The heating sequence begins with two series of 5 pulses – the first series at the initial position and the second series 1 cm below. Five pulses are used in the initial two sequences as the first two pulses of the five are not good quality steam as the catheter needs to heat up to aid thermal diffusion. Once started, the catheter is withdrawn one centimetre at a time. At each centimetre, 3 or 4 pulses are applied depending on the mean size of the vein:
- 3 pulses if the vein is up to 7 mm
- 4 pulses for larger veins

For localized dilatations, 5 pulses can be used without adverse consequences. Additional cooling around the entry point is needed to avoid skin burns here and injecting tumescence fluid around this area is sufficient. At the end of the procedure a compressive bandage is applied, it can be replaced by stockings when the patient leaves the clinic.

Treating Tributaries and Recurrent Varicose Veins

The Trib-Vein® catheter fires forward to allow steam to cross convoluted varicosities (Figure 2). However, once one vein is heated, the other superficial veins often go into spasm. Thus it is necessary to put all the introducers in place before beginning to heat any of the veins. The introducers used for this part of the operation are 18 G venous cannulae (Green) and ultrasound guidance is used to ensure accurate placement (Figure 3).

Once all of the introducers are in place, the heating Trib-Vein® catheter is introduced into each in turn. Tumescent anaesthesia is applied in small quantities around the veins to be treated (Figure 4) and the skin is cooled by placing gauze "swabs" impregnated with ice-cold saline onto the skin over the area to be treated. Heating is achieved by a series of 3 pulses under ultrasound control. Using the ultrasound, we can visualise the extent of steam diffusion and the efficacy of the treatment. When the vein becomes non compressible the desired result has been achieved. From our experience, we advise that 12 pulses per puncture point is the maximum treatment per area.

Immediately after heating, more tumescence fluid is injected over the whole area. This helps to cool the tissues and compress the treated vein to minimize the size of the thrombus, thus limiting pigmentation and inflammatory reactions.

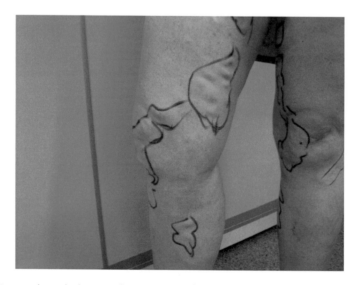

Figure 3: Markings made on the legs to indicate position of varicose veins and where the introducers need to be positioned (recurrent varicose veins).

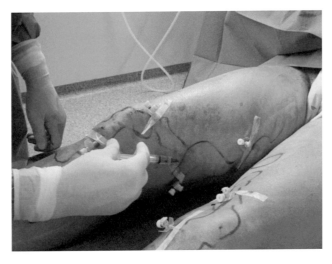

Figure 4: Introducers in place and local anaesthetic being administered prior to heating.

Treating Incompetent Perforators

The Flexi-Vein® catheter with lateral holes is used in the treatment of incompetent perforating veins (IPV). The incompetent perforator is punctured with a 16 G intravenous cannula. The heating catheter is advanced into the perforator under ultrasound guidance, if possible, just at the level of the deep fascia. Tumescent anaesthesia is injected around the catheter tip. Five pulses are emitted and the catheter is withdrawn 1 cm. A further 5 pulses are then emitted from this position. We have found that this treatment regime is usually enough to close an incompetent perforating vein. The risk of DVT is minimal as only droplets of hot water enter the deep veins and the faster flow in the deep veins rapidly dissipates the heat.

Treating Venous Malformations

Large trunks such as the Marginal veins seen in Klippel Trenaunay syndrome can be occluded successfully using the Flexi-Vein® catheter and the same technique as we use for the saphenous trunks. We have found it necessary to use more heat in these veins than we would do for a same calibre saphenous trunk and we have used up to 10 pulses per cm. It is thus mandatory to apply a larger quantity of tumescence fluid and to stop heating every 60 pulses to let the heat dissipate. We use a 15 second pause after every 60 pulses. Post-operatively a long duration (6 weeks) of anticoagulation is necessary as these patients are prone to major thrombo-embolic complications. Localized malformations are treated with the Trib Vein® catheter.

Results

Pilot Clinical Studies

2 pilot clinical studies were performed.

We performed our first study in 2007, treating 10 Great Saphenous Veins in 9 patients aged 36 to

65 years. The patients were treated under general anaesthesia with tumescence fluid injected around the vein under ultrasound guidance. One skin burn was observed because the hot catheter remained in contact with unprotected skin. No DVTs, PEs or infections were reported. Pain level was low and no post-operative pain-killers were given. At the 3 months control all vein were closed. At 1 year one vein was partially opened above knee and at 2 years, 8 veins were checked and 2 showed partial re-opening.

A second study was performed in the Rotterdam Erasmus Medical Center[3]. Twenty patients were treated under tumescent anaesthesia alone. No major adverse incidents were reported. Ecchymosis was seen in 9 patients and one had phlebitis of the vein segment distal to the entry point. Mean pain score was 1.8 on an analogue scale of 0 to 10 (0 being no pain and 10 being the worst pain possible) and patient's satisfaction rated at 9.25 on the same 10 point analogue scale (10 being perfectly satisfied). At 6 months check-up, 13 veins were totally occluded, 5 had a patent segment without reflux and 2 a refluxing segment. These veins were treated at 1 pulse/cm, which had been shown to be insufficient in the previous *in-vitro* studies described above.

French Multi-Centre Study

A multi-centre study was performed in 4 centres from 2008 to 2010 and published in 2012 in the European Journal of Vascular and Endovascular Surgery[4]. Seventy-five patients with GSV insufficiency were treated, 92% had sapheno-femoral insufficiency and 73% reflux down to the mid-calf level. The mean length treated was 42 cm. The primary endpoint was obliteration of the full length of the vein and this was achieved in 96% of patients. The secondary endpoint was the absence of reflux at 1 year and this was observed in 92 % of patients. No significant or lasting adverse event was reported. One patient had a skin burn at the entry point of the catheter due to defective cooling of the skin. Pain level was low, only 5 patients reported a pain over 5 on an analogue scale of 0 to 10. The median post-operative pain level was 0.75 on the same scale.

Tributary study: Foam versus Steam, randomized study

In 2011, we presented a randomized study comparing steam obliteration and foam sclerotherapy for treating large tributaries in 20 patients[5] at the American College of Phlebology meeting. Aethoxysclerol 1% was used as the sclerosant and foam was made using the Tessari method. Eight days after treatment, pain and inflammation were significantly lower in the steam group – 0.5 for pain and 2.4 for inflammation reported in 6 patients after foam sclerotherapy and 0 for both after steam treatment. At the 1 month follow up, skin pigmentation was reported in 12 patients after foam and 4 after steam. At 3 months all treated segments were closed in both groups.

Conclusion

Mid-term results of steam obliteration are comparable to those reported after other endovenous thermoablation techniques and will be improved now that dose-finding has been completed. The safety profile is very good with low levels of post-operative pain. The main advantage of steam lies in the possibility to treat not only saphenous trunks, but recurrences and large subcutaneous varicose veins without incision.

The potential complications of foam sclerotherapy of allergic reactions and neurologic problems related to air embolism are avoided when using steam obliteration for large varicose veins. The equipment is less expensive than some other endovenous thermoablation system and if research confirms the cost savings for the whole treatment, steam may allow more patients to benefit from endovenous thermal ablation.

References

1. Proebstle T. Lehr HA, Kargl A et al. treatment of the Great saphenous vein with a 940mm diode laser: thrombotic occlusion after endoluminal thermal damage generated by steam bubbles. J Vasc Surg. 2002; 35: 729-36

2. Van den Bos R, Arends L, Kockaert M, Neumann M, Nijsten T. Endovenous therapies of lower extremity varicosities: a meta-analysis. J Vasc Surg. 2009; 49: 230-9

3. Van den Bos RR, Milleret R, Neumann M, Nijsten T. Proof-of-principle study of steam ablation as novel thermal therapy for saphenous varicose veins. J Vasc Surg. 2011; 53: 181–4

4. Milleret R, Huot L, Nicolini P, Creton D, Roux AS, Decullier E, Chapuis FR, Camelot G. Great saphenous vein ablation with steam injection: results of a multicentre study. Eur J Vasc Endovasc Surg. 2013;45 (4):391-6.

5. Milleret R. Randomised Comparative study of ablation of varicose veins with steam and foam. American College of Phlebology meeting. Los Angeles - Nov 2011

Chapter 10

Mechanochemical ablation of varicose veins – an update on a non-tumescence technique

Author(s)
Doeke Boersma[1,2]
Ramon RJP van Eekeren[3]
Michel MPJ Reijnen[3]
Jean-Paul PM de Vries[4]

Institution(s)
(1) Department of Surgery, Jeroen Bosch Ziekenhuis, Den Bosch, The Netherlands
(2) Department of Vascular Surgery, University Medical Centre Utrecht, Utrecht, The Netherlands
(3) Department of Surgery, Rijnstate Hospital, Arnhem, The Netherlands
(4) Department of Vascular Surgery, St. Antonius Hospital, Nieuwegein, The Netherlands

Introduction

Venous insufficiency of the lower extremities is a common condition and is related to various symptoms, including venous ulcers. The effect of venous insufficiency on patients' health-related quality of life is substantial and comparable with other chronic diseases such as arthritis, diabetes, and cardiovascular disease[1]. Superficial venous reflux, to a greater or lesser extent, will develop in approximately 40% of women and 20% of men during their lifetime[2]. These problems are mostly associated with insufficiency of great saphenous veins (GSVs); however, insufficiency of the small saphenous vein (SSV) is responsible for complaints in 15% of patients with varicose veins[3]. Until the 1990s, high ligation combined with surgical stripping was the gold standard in the treatment of GSV insufficiency, whereas standard of care in (surgical) treatment of SSV insufficiency was lacking.

The introduction of minimally invasive therapies has revolutionized the treatment of varicose veins. Chemical ablation, in which foam or liquid sclerotherapy is administered, is a widely used technique for truncal and reticular veins. Endothermal catheter modalities, including endovenous laser ablation (EVLA) and radiofrequency ablation (RFA), have become preferred techniques due to excellent success rates in both GSV and SSV[4,5]. In these techniques, the insufficient vein is ablated by heating the venous wall, but heat-related complications, such as prolonged pain, skin burns, and nerve injury, may occur despite tumescent anaesthesia[4-7].

Mechanochemical endovenous ablation (MOCA), using the ClariVein catheter (Vascular Insights, Madison, CT, USA), is a recently introduced treatment with a unique working mechanism. MOCA combines mechanical injury to the venous endothelium with simultaneous delivery and dispersion of sclerosant. Because no heat is generated during MOCA therapy, tumescent anaesthesia is no longer needed and thermal injury cannot occur.

ClariVein

The concept of mechanochemical endovenous ablation and the ClariVein device were developed in 2005 by the interventional radiologist Michael Tal. During his work, he was confronted by patients with varicosities in which thermal ablation and foam sclerotherapy were both contraindicated. In animal experiments, Tal observed that the combination of mechanical injury with liquid sclerotherapy had superior results compared with both components individually. The best occlusion rate in these experiments was seen with the current design, which consists of an angle dispersion wire with a ball-shaped end. Selected data from these animal experiments were published in 2015[8]. The ClariVein system is a single-use, disposable, two-component device: the catheter unit and the motor unit. The two components are distributed together in a sealed and sterilized package. The sclerosant is infused through the catheter unit, which consists of a 2.67F (0.89-mm diameter) catheter available in a length of 45 or 65 cm. A stainless steel wire is fitted within the lumen of the catheter. This dispersion wire has an angled tip with a small ball fitted to the end. When the components are disconnected, the catheter covers the angled tip. The catheter and wire are connected to a plastic base with a 3-way Luer-Lock port (Figure 1a).

The 9-volt battery-powered motor unit is a white plastic handpiece. Once the two parts are connected, the wire tip protrudes from the catheter (Figure 1b), and the motor can rotate the dispersion wire in various speeds, ranging from 2000 to 3500 rotations per minute (rpm). A plastic holding clip is used to connect a 5-mL syringe to the Luer-Lock port. This syringe is used for flushing the system and infusing the sclerosing agent. When the device is connected, the hand piece

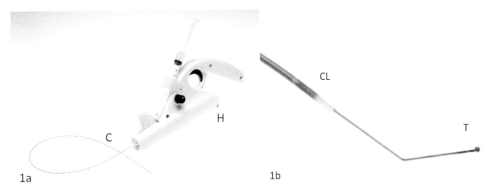

Figure 1: (a) ClariVein device consists of motor unit (H) and infusion catheter (C). (b) The unsheathed dispersion tip (T) protrudes with angulated tip from catheter (CL).

allows steering the device, activating the motor by compressing the trigger with the index finger, and controlling simultaneous infusion of sclerosant with the thumb on the syringe.

Treatment

<u>Preparation</u>

In the current (study) protocols, no preoperative analgesics, anticoagulants, or antibiotics are administered. The liquid sclerosant is prepared in the chosen concentration.

The ClariVein catheter is taken from the sterile package. The side port to the 3-way valve is capped with a stopcock, and the system is flushed with sterile saline. The valve is closed by turning the handle 45° to avoid blood leak and clot in between the catheter and the metal wire during insertion of the device into the vein. Flushing the system with sclerosant is not advised due to the risk of clotting inside the catheter. The battery of the motor unit is checked. A small light-emitting diode is activated when the trigger is pulled. The switch is set to the maximum speed of 3500 rpm. The motor will not start until both units are connected.

<u>Access and placement</u>

The procedure to obtain percutaneous access to the varicose vein is similar to other endovenous techniques. Duplex ultrasound examination is used to plan the point of access distal to the insufficient part of the vein. A major advantage of the MOCA technique is that local anaesthesia is only needed at the point of access. The patient is positioned supine with a cushion under the knee to enhance access to the medial part of the thigh when the GSV is insufficient or is positioned facedown when the SSV is treated. Ultrasound guidance is used to puncture the vein with an 18-gauge needle. A 4F sheath is introduced over a short guidewire.

The ClariVein catheter can be introduced via the sheath, without any additional guidewire. The tip of the catheter is placed with ultrasound guidance at the planned location. Owing to the small calibre of the ClariVein device and the slightly angled tip of the sheath tip, it is easy to steer and position. A

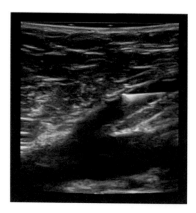

Figure 2: Ultrasound image shows the ball-shaped wire tip is positioned in the proximal great saphenous vein.

small plastic wing is attached to the base of the catheter unit to optimize rotatory steer-ability. When the catheter is placed in the proximal GSV or SSV, the wire tip is unsheathed by connecting the catheter and motor unit. To optimize safety, it is very important to visualize the ball shaped tip of the wire at the planned position (Figure 2). When the ball at the tip cannot be visualized, it should be assumed that the tip is placed too proximal, which risks injury to the deep venous system and deep venous thrombosis (DVT).

In the early experience, the tip was placed 2 cm distally from the saphenofemoral junction (SFJ). With growing experience, the distance between tip and the SFJ has been shortened or just distal to the orifice of the superficial epigastric vein. In the more recent Dutch studies, the tip was positioned only 0.5 cm distal to the SFJ. For SSV ablation, the manufacturer advises positioning the tip distal to the fascial curve or 2 cm distal to insertion of the gastrocnemius vein.

Procedure

Adequate placement of the tip is rechecked after the catheter and motor-unit are connected and the 5-mL syringe filled with sclerosant is attached. The motor is activated by pulling the trigger. The rotating tip will induce spasm to the proximal part of the vein. To obtain spasm, the motor is activated for 5-10 seconds without movement or infusion of sclerosant. The spasm is considered important to prevent leakage of sclerosant into the deep veins. The activated device is then pulled back 1 cm every 7 seconds. The sclerosant is administered simultaneously (Figure 3). Even though no tumescent anaesthesia is injected, pain has hardly been reported during the procedure, and some

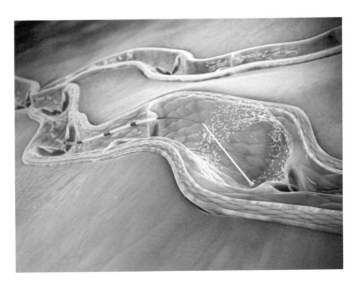

Figure 3: The ClariVein device is placed in the planned position in the target vein. By connecting the catheter and the motor unit, the dispersion tip is unsheathed. The syringe filled with sclerosant is attached. After induction of vasospasm solely by mechanical action of the rotating tip, the activated device is pulled back and simultaneous infusion of sclerosant is controlled by operating the attached syringe. Acknowledgement: Figure 3 is reproduced with permission from Vascular Insights, LCC

patients describe a tickling sensation. Directly after the procedure, the patient is asked to flex and extend the foot to let the calf muscle pump clear any sclerosant from the deep venous system. As with other endovenous ablation techniques, patients are recommended to walk immediately after the completion of MOCA. Patients are discharged with class 2 compression stockings (30-40 mm Hg) and advised to wear these continuously during the first 24 hours and during the daytime for the following 1-2 weeks.

Follow-up is planned 4 to 6 weeks after treatment to determine clinical success and duplex ultrasound assessment is used to show anatomical success. At this point, additional phlebectomies or sclerotherapy can be planned. In patients not included in clinical studies, the need for further follow-up after successful treatment can be debated.

Sclerotherapy

Two types of sclerosant are used in clinical studies. In the studies from the United Kingdom, United States of America, and Australia, sodium tetradecyl sulphate (STS) (trademarks: Sotradecol, Bioniche Pharma Group, Geneva, Switzerland or Fibrovein, STD Pharmaceuticals, Hereford, UK) was infused in a 1.5% or 2% concentration. In the Dutch studies, polidocanol (trademark: Aethoxysklerol, Kreussler Pharma, Wiesbaden, Germany) was used in different concentrations. In an initial safety study, 1.5% polidocanol was administered. In an attempt to optimize technical success, the proximal part of the vein was treated with 2% polidocanol and the rest of the vein with a concentration of 1.5%.

The amount of sclerosant used is determined by the diameter and length of treated veins. A dosing table published by the manufacturer is available as a guideline. It is important not to exceed the maximum allowed daily dosage, due to the possible side effects of the sclerosant.

Patient Selection

The current studies give no explicit guideline for patient selection. The majority of patients included have long-segment incompetent GSVs and SSVs with diameters ranging from 3 to 12 mm. No series of MOCA in larger diameters have been published so far. The mechanical effect on larger veins may be diminished by the 6.5-mm radius of the dispersion wire. As in other endovenous techniques, severe tortuosity may be considered an exclusion criterion. In general, a vein considered adequate for any other endovenous therapy is also accessible for MOCA. Although all published data consist of long-segment GSV and SSV, our experience is that MOCA is a technically feasible and effective treatment of short, anterolateral, and even perforating branches. In addition, Mueller et al.[9] published tips and tricks on treating miscellaneous varicosities.

Patients with allergies or any other contraindication to the sclerosant, history of ipsilateral deep venous thrombosis, coagulation disorders, or severe peripheral arterial disease are considered unsuitable for MOCA. There is no definitive data on either safety or teratogenic effects of STS or polidocanol and therefore MOCA is discouraged during pregnancy.

	Eekeren 2011[10]	Elias 2012[11]	Boersma 2013[12]	Vun 2015[13]	Bishawi/ Kim 2014/2016[14,15]	Deijen 2016[16]	Lam 2016[17]		Bootun / Lane 2014/2016[18,19]	Tang 2016[20]	Eekeren/ Witte 2014/2016[21,22]
							Liquid	Microfoam			
Country	Netherlands	USA	Netherlands	Australia	USA	Netherlands	Netherlands	Netherlands	UK	UK	Netherlands
Study design	P	P	P	n/a	P	n/a	RCT	RCT	RCT	P	P
Population											
Total	30	30	50	57	126	570	53	23	83	393	106
GSV	30	30	0	51	126	438	53	23	77	333	106
SSV	0	0	50	6	0	132	0	0	6	60	0
Sclerosant	POL 1.5%	STS 1.5%	POL 2% / 1.5%	STS 1.5%	STS or POL	POL 2% / 1.5%	POL 2 or 3%	POL 1% microfoam	STS 2.0%	STS 2.0%	POL 2% / 1.5%
Technical success, %	100	100	100	n/a	100	98	n/a	n/a	n/a	100	99
Anatomic success, n (%)											
up to 8 weeks	29/30 (96)	29/30 (96)	50/50 (100)	52/57 (91)	126/126 (100)	457/506 (90)^	46/53 (87)	7/23 (30)	64/69 (93)	382/393 (97)	n/a
6 months	n/a	29/30 (96)	n/a	n/a	84/89 (94)	n/a	n/a	n/a	54/62 (87)	n/a	96/103 (93)
1 year	n/a	n/a	44/47 (94)	n/a	75/79 (95)	n/a	n/a	n/a	n/a	n/a	90/102 (88)
2 years	n/a	n/a	n/a	n/a	60/65 (92)	n/a	n/a	n/a	n/a	n/a	64/71(90)
3 years	n/a	n/a	n/a	n/a	n/a	n/a	n/a	n/a	n/a	n/a	42/48(87)^^
Clinical success											
VCSS	3 ⟶ 1*	n/a	3 ⟶ 1*	n/a	9.5 ⟶ 3*	n/a	6 ⟶ 3*		5 ⟶ 2*	n/a	4 ⟶ 1*
Major complications	none	none	none	n/a	none	2 PE / 2 DVT / 1 paraesthesia	none		1 DVT	none	none

P, prospective cohort; RCT, randomized controlled trial; GSV, great saphenous vein; SSV, short saphenous vein; n/a not available; VCSS, Venous Clinical Severity Score; DVT, deep venous thrombosis; PE pulmonary embolism. ‡two publications on same patient population; ^median follow up of 54 days (range 12 - 266 days) / anatomical success 92% in GSV / 87% in SSV; ^^median follow up of 36 months (range 12.5 – 46.3 days) ;*statistically significant

Table 1. Overview of results MOCA in published clinical studies

Results

Clinical data

Since Food and Drug Administration (FDA) approval in the United States in 2008 and Conformité Européene (CE) marking in Europe in 2010, several clinical studies have been conducted and published. Table 1 provides a complete overview of all published clinical data on MOCA[10-22].

Safety studies

The first two studies focussed on feasibility and safety of the MOCA treatment and ClariVein device. The first to present and later publish their data were Elias et al. They treated 29 patients with GSV insufficiency in 30 limbs using the ClariVein catheter and Sotradecol 1.5%. The primary objectives were to determine overall safety of MOCA and the primary closure rate at 6 months. No major complications, defined as DVT, nerve injury or skin burn, were seen, and minor ecchymosis occurred in 10%. The anatomic success rate was 97% (29/30) at 6 months. Clinical success was not described[11].

After introduction of the ClariVein device in Europe in 2010, a collaborative venous study group in the Netherlands were the first to publish a prospective observational study which included 30 consecutive GSVs in 25 patients. Polidocanol was used in a 1.5% concentration. The main objectives were to evaluate technical feasibility and safety. Clinical and anatomic success were evaluated at 6 weeks of follow-up. To measure clinical success, the Venous Clinical Severity Score (VCSS) was assessed before treatment and after 6 weeks.

MOCA was technically feasible in all patients. Anatomical success was achieved in 29/30 limbs. Full recanalisation occurred in 1 limb. No major complications occurred. Local ecchymosis and hematoma at the puncture site were seen in up to 30%. Clinical success was illustrated by a significant decrease in VCSS from 3.0 (interquartile range, 2.0-4.75) to 1.0 (interquartile range, 0.25-3.0;P<.001)[10].

Clinical cohorts and trials

Including the two safety studies described above, 13 clinical papers encompassing 10 cohorts were published from The Netherlands (5), United Kingdom (2), USA (2) and Australia (1). All study results are depicted in Table 1. Three patient cohorts were described in 2 serial publications, and the data on these cohort were extracted from both publications and combined. In total 1521 veins were treated with MOCA and analysed. In 5 cohorts polidocanol was used, in 4 STS, and in 1 both sclerosants were used in different concentrations. Immediate technical success was 99%. Anatomical success is 93, 92, 91 and 87% after 6 months, 1 year, 2 and 3 years respectively. Although these results suggest a long-lasting anatomical success rate around 90%, it should be appreciated that the number of cases with follow-up over 1 year is limited and "lost-to-follow-up" is significant.

The first and only study solely focussing on MOCA in SSV was published in 2012 and included 50 consecutive patients with primary long-segment SSV insufficiency. The first 15 patients were treated with polidocanol 1.5%. In the following 35 patients, 2% polidocanol was used to treat the proximal 10 to 15 cm and 1.5% was used to treat the remainder of the vein. Initial occlusion and anatomic success at 6 weeks were obtained in all 50 patients. At the 1-year follow-up, the overall anatomic success was 94%, comprising 87% in the 1.5% group and 97% in 2% group (NS)[12]. Deijen et al. included within their very large cohort of 570 veins a total of 132 SSVs. Within this subgroup, they report an anatomical success rate of 85% and 80.5% after 6 weeks and 3 months respectively (although lost to follow-up was not mentioned)[16].

Clinical success and pain scores were comparable with results from GSV studies.

The pooled data underline that MOCA is a safe treatment modality. Major complications are extremely rare. Deep venous thrombosis were seen in 0.3% and pulmonary embolism in 0.2%. Only 1 case of transient paraesthesia was reported in a pooled cohort of 1464 treated veins. This is a clinically important message, especially in treating SSVs and GSVs below the knee.

Pain studies

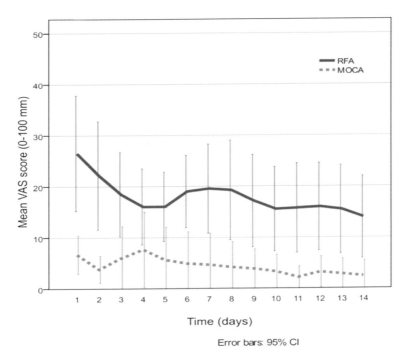

Figure 4: Mean postoperative pain scores on a 0- to 100-mm visual analogue scale (VAS) during 14 days after mechanochemical ablation (MOCA) and radiofrequency ablation (RFA). Acknowledgement: Figure 4 is reprinted from Journal of Vascular Surgery 2013, with permission from Elsevier[12].

In 2012, Van Eekeren et al. published a prospective observational study in the Journal of Vascular Surgery on pain and health-related quality of life (HR-QoL) after MOCA compared with RFA. The study included 68 patients with unilateral GSV insufficiency, of which 34 were treated with MOCA and the other half with RFA (VNUS ClosureFast, VNUS Medical Technologies, Sunnyvale, CA, USA). Pain scores in the MOCA group during the 2 weeks after treatment were significantly lower in MOCA compared with RFA (Figure 4). Pain scores during treatment and complications were not significantly different between the groups in this study. Clinical symptoms (VCSS) and HR-QoL improved in both groups (NS)[23].

Bootun et al. reported on intraprocedural pain scores in a larger RCT, randomizing 119 legs between MOCA (60) and RFA (59) using Venefit (Covidien, San Jose, CA, USA). The mean VAS pain score during treatment was significantly lower in MOCA (2.6±2.2) compared to RFA (4.4±2.7) (P=.001). Maximum procedural pain scores were also significantly lower in MOCA. In line with the study above, the clinical and HR-QoL improved in both groups (NS)[18].

Experimental data

The working mechanism of MOCA is becoming more and more elucidated, due to the following experimental studies.

In 2015 Tal et al., partially disclosed the data on the initial animal experiments by the manufacturing company. These results are very valuable, because they described the tissue reaction in a standardized model up to 12 weeks after MOCA. Duplex ultrasound showed occlusion in MOCA treated veins. All veins in the control groups (ClariVein without sclerosant or solely liquid sclerotherapy) remained fully patent. After MOCA, microscopy showed complete occlusion, wall thickening with endothelial injury and extensive fibrotic changes of the vein[8].

A more recent large animal study, including 18 goats was conducted, focusing on tissue reaction after MOCA, mechanical injury and liquid sclerotherapy in both the acute and follow up setting. This acute experiments prove the hypothesis that MOCA improves the potency of liquid sclerosant by inducing (limited) endothelial injury combined with a distinct vasoconstrictive effect. The endothelial injury might lead to easier penetration of the vein wall, and vasoconstriction increase the effect of, sclerosant by decreasing dilution of sclerosants and prolonging exposure of it to the vein wall. In the follow up experiments occlusion was only found in MOCA treated veins, the occlusion due to organized thrombus formation and fibrotic changes. All veins in the control groups remained patent[24].

Van Eekeren et al. are unique in describing histology of a human vein explanted 1 year after successful MOCA treatment. This vein was completely obliterated and histologically examined. In line with two animal studies described above, the microscopy revealed total disappearance of the endothelium with fibrotic neo-intima proliferation. The damage extended well into the media layer[26].

Discussion

This chapter provides an overview of all published results of MOCA in GSV and SSV. Initial technical success was 99%, and at short-term follow-up, the anatomic success was 94%. Mid-term results range from 87 to 96% and anatomical success rates after 2 to 3 years stabilize at 87 to 91%.

Perhaps even more important are the good clinical success rates observed with MOCA. In all 8 studies (6 cohorts), describing the clinical symptoms of varicose disease before and after treatment, a significant decrease in VCSS was measured[10, 12, 14, 15, 17-19, 21, 22]. In addition, studies repeatedly showed that MOCA treatment led to a significant improvement in HR-QoL (without significant difference compared with RFA)[18, 19, 21-23].

An interesting observation was the difference in anatomic success between the two groups in the SSV study: the first group was treated with 1.5% polidocanol, and the second was treated with 2% polidocanol in the proximal section. The difference was not significant, probably because of the small number of patients, but an elevated dosage of liquid sclerosant may be key in further optimizing anatomic occlusion rates in MOCA[12]. All studies afterwards used increased concentrations of polidocanol. A large dose-finding RCT is still enrolling patients at this moment, comparing 3 groups: MOCA with 2% liquid polidocanol, MOCA with 3% liquid polidocanol and MOCA with 1% polidocanol microfoam (off label use). An interim analysis revealed that results after MOCA with use of microfoam were abominable (only 30% anatomical success) and this treatment modality was removed from the RCT[17]. Until final results of this RCT are published, there will be no definitive answer on the question of whether increasing concentration leads to improved results.

Furthermore, it is up for discussion which is the optimal sclerosant to be used in MOCA: although STS has been shown to be a more potent sclerosant than polidocanol (*in-vitro*)[26], there are no studies conducted so far comparing MOCA with the different agents. Randomized controlled studies between different sclerosing agents might be difficult because in some countries, STS and polidocanol are not both registered for this indication.

A clinically relevant advantage of MOCA is that only local anaesthesia at the puncture site is necessary instead of tumescent anaesthesia. Administering tumescent anaesthesia is not only a painful burden to the patients, due to multiple injections, but is also time-consuming, leading to a shorter duration of treatment in MOCA compared with other endothermal ablation techniques[23]. Patient-reported pain during and in the weeks after treatment is significantly less in the MOCA compared to RFA[18,19,23].

All treatment modalities of varicose veins have their specific complications. Especially in SSV treatment, the anatomic proximity of the sural nerve poses an additional risk. Endothermal ablation of SSVs lead to paraesthesia in 4.8% (EVLA) to 9.7% (RFA)[5]. Pooled data showed that the risk of (transient) paraesthesia after MOCA is less than 0.1%. Other major complications, such as DVT and pulmonary embolism, also occur only rarely (0.1 – 0.2%).

With the constantly increasing number of studies published on the results of MOCA on GSV and SSV insufficiency, it could be stated MOCA is already a proven alternative to endothermal ablation. Especially, due to the fact that no tumescence is necessary and as MOCA has significantly lower pain scores compared to endothermal ablation, MOCA should be considered an important treatment option. Nevertheless, there are some limitations. Firstly: all published data are either cohort studies or RCTs not powered for anatomical success. Unfortunately, the randomized controlled trial for treatment of the SSV was stopped after inclusion of only a small number of patients[27] and the RCT comparing MOCA and RFA in the treatment of the GSV stopped recruitment prematurely[28]. Secondly, the data relating to long-term anatomical success rates is limited and subject to a large number of patients lost-to-follow up. Finally, there is still only limited information available as to which is the better sclerosant for use in MOCA and what the optimal dosing is.

Conclusion
Mechanochemical endovenous ablation using the ClariVein® device has proven itself to be an innovative tumescent-less technique for treating great and small saphenous venous insufficiency. The anatomic and clinical success rates can compete with results of current endothermal techniques, whereas important downsides to thermal ablation, such as tumescent anaesthesia, pain, and nerve injury, seem to be history.

References

1. Andreozzi GM, Cordova RM, Scomparin A, Martini R, D'Eri A, Andreozzi F; Quality of Life Working Group on Vascular Medicine of SIAPAV. Quality of life in chronic venous insufficiency. An Italian pilot study of the Triveneto Region. Int Angiol. 2005;24:272-7.

2. Callam MJ. Epidemiology of varicose veins. Br J Surg. 1994;81:167-173.

3. Almgren B, Eriksson E. Valvular incompetence in superficial, deep and perforator veins of limbs with varicose veins. Acta Chirurg Scand. 1990;156:69–74.

4. Van den Bos R, Arends L, Kockaert M, Neumann M, Nijsten T. Endovenous therapy of lower extremity varicosities: a meta-analysis. J Vasc Surg. 2009;49:230-9.

5. Boersma D, Kornmann VN, Eekeren RR, Tromp E, Unlu C, Reijnen MM, De Vries JP. Treatment modalities for small saphenous vein insufficiency: Systematic review and meta-analysis. J Endovasc Ther. 2016; 23: 199-211.

6. Van den Bos RR, Neumann M, De Roos KP, NijstenT. Endovenous laser ablation-induced complications: review of literature and new cases. Dermatol Surg. 2009;35:1206-14.

7. Sichlau MJ, Ryu RK. Cutaneous thermal injury after endovenous laser ablation of the great saphenous vein. J Vasc Interv Radiol. 2004; 15: 865-7

8. Tal MG, Dos Santos SJ, Marano JP, Whiteley MS. Histologic findings after mechanochemical ablation in a caprine model with use of ClariVein. J Vasc Surg: Venous Lymphat Disord. 2015; 3: 81-5

9. Mueller RL, Raines JK. ClariVein Mechanochemical Ablation Background and Procedural Details. Vasc Endovasc Surg. 2013;47:195-206.

10. Van Eekeren RRJP, Boersma D, Elias S, Holewijn S, Werson DAB, De Vries JPPM, Reijnen MMJP. Endovenous mechanochemical Ablation of great saphenous vein incompetence using the ClariVein device: a safety study. J Endovasc Ther. 2011;18:328-334

11. Elias S, Raines JK. Mechanochemical tumescentless endovenous ablation: final results of the initial clinical trial. Phlebology. 2012;27:67-72.

12. Boersma D, Van Eekeren RRJP, Werson DAB, Reijnen MMJP, De Vries JPPM. Mechanochemical endovenous ablation of small saphenous vein insufficiency using the ClariVein® device: One-year results of a prospective series. Eur J Vasc Endovasc Surg. 2013;45:299-303

13. Vun SV, Rashid ST, Blst NC, Spark JI. Lower pain and faster treatment with mechano-chemical endovenous ablation using ClariVein. Phlebology. 2015;30:688-92.

14. Bishawi M, Bernstein R, Boter M, Draughn D, Gould CF, Hamilton C, Koziarski J. Mechano-chemical ablation in patients with chronic venous disease: a prospective multicenter report. Phlebology. 2014; 29: 397–400.

15. Kim PS, Bishawi M, Draughn D, Boter M, Gould CF, Koziarski J, Bernstein R, Hamilton C. Mechanochemical ablation for symptomatic great saphenous vein reflux: a two-year follow up. Phlebology 2016 ePub ahead of print.

16. Deijen CL, Schreve MA, Bosma J, De Nie AJ, Leijdekkers VJ, Van den Akker PJ, Vahl A. Clarivein mechanochemical ablation of the great and small saphenous vein: early treatment

outcomes of two hospitals. Phlebology. 2016;31:192-7.

17. Lam YL, Toonder IM, Wittens CHA. ClariVein mechano-chemical ablation an interim analysis of a randomized controlled trial dose-finding study. Phlebology 2016;31:170-6.

18. Bootun R, Lane T, Dharmarajah B, Lim CS, Najem M, Renton S, Sritharan K, Davies AH. Intra-procedural pain score in a randomised controlled trial comparing mechanochemical ablation to radiofrequency ablation: the Multicentre Venefit versus ClariVein for varicose veins trial. Phlebology. 2016;31:61-5

19. Lane T, Bootun R, Dharmarajah B, Lim CS, Najem M, Renton S, Sritharan K, Davies AH. A multi-centre randomised controlled trial comparingradiofrequency and mechanical occlusion chemically assited ablation of varicose veins - final results of the Venefit versus ClariVein for varicose veins trial. Phlebology 2016 ePub ahead of print.

20. Tang TY, Kam JW, Gaunt ME. ClariVein - Early results of a large single centre series of mechanochemical endovenous ablation for varicose veins. Phlebology 2016 ePub ahead of print.

21. Van Eekeren RRJP, Boersma D, Holewijn S, Werson DAB, De Vries JPPM, Reijnen MMJP. Mechanochemical endovenous ablation for the treatment of great saphenous vein insufficiency. J Vasc Surg Venous Lymphat Disord. 2014;2:282-8

22. Witte ME, Holewijn S, Van Eekeren RR, De Vries JP, Zeebregts CJ, Reijnen MMPJ Reijnen. Mid-term outcome of mechanochemical endovenous ablation for the treatment of great saphenous vein insuffiency. J EndoVasc Ther. 2016; 24 (1): 149-155.

23. Van Eekeren RRJP, Boersma D, Konijn V, De Vries JPPM, Reijnen MMJP. Postoperative pain and early quality of life after radiofrequency ablation and mechanochemical endovenous ablation of incompetent great saphenous veins. J Vasc Surg. 2013;57:445-50

24. Boersma D, Van Haelst STW, Van Eekeren RRJP, Vink A, Reijnen MMJP, De Vries JPPM, De Borst GJ. Macroscopic and histologic analysis of vessel wall reaction after mechanochemical endovenous ablation using the ClariVein OC device in an animal model. EJVES. 2017; 53(2): 290-298.

25. van Eekeren RR, Hillebrands JL, van der Sloot K, de Vries JP, Zeebregts CJ, Reijnen MM. Histological observations one year after mechanochemical endovenous ablation of the great saphenous vein. J Endovasc Ther. 2014;21(3):429-33

26. McAreeB, Ikponmwosa A, Brockbank K, Abbott C, Homer-Vanniasinkam S, Gough MJ. Comparative stability of sodium tetradecylsulphate (STD) and polidocanol foam: impact on vein damage in an *in-vitro* model. Eur J Vasc Endovasc Surg. 2012;43:721– 5.

27. Boersma D, Van Eekeren RRJP, Kelder JC, Werson DAB, Holewijn S, Schreve MA, Reijnen MMPJ, De Vries JPPM. Mechanochemical endovenous ablation versus radiofrequency ablation in the treatment of primary small saphenous vein insufficiency (MESSI trial): study protocol for a randomized controlled trial Trials. 2014;15:421

28. Van Eekeren RRJP, Boersma D, Holewijn S, Vahl A, De Vries JPPM, Zeebregts CJ, Reijnen MMPJ. Mechanochemical endovenous Ablation versus RADiOfrequeNcy Ablation in the

treatment of primary great saphenous vein incompetence (MARADONA): study protocol for a randomized controlled trial Trials. 2014;15:121

Chapter 11

Cyanoacrylate Adhesive – a new technique in the treatment of varicose veins without tumescent local anaesthesia and without compression treatment

Author
Thomas M. Proebstle

Institution(s)
(1) Dept.of Dermatology, University Medical Center, Mainz, Germany
(2) Private Clinic Proebstle, Mannheim, Germany

Introduction
For more than a decade, various techniques for endothermal ablation of incompetent veins have evolved. These include lasers of various near-infrared wavelengths using different types of aiming lights, a variety of radiofrequency powered systems and also the use of superheated pressurized steam. All these technologies have registered CE marks in Europe and have proved to be safe and effective for the endovenous ablation of incompetent saphenous veins and their larger tributaries as well as, in most instances, ablation of incompetent perforating veins. Because of their short period of convalescence with less pain and morbidity when compared to classic surgery, they allow early return to work and early return to normal physical activity. Therefore, the Society for Vascular Surgery and the American Venous Forum clinical practice guidelines have ranked endovenous thermal ablation (EVTA) over traditional high ligation and stripping surgery[1]. Nevertheless, despite high venous occlusion rates with limited downtime[2-4], thermal ablation requires

- the placement of perivenous tumescent anesthesia
- the use of postinterventional compression therapy as standard care
- and has the potential for perivenous tissue damage resulting in post-operative pain, bruising and other complications like sensory nerve damage[5,6].

Before the appearance of Cyanoacrylate (CA) adhesive, all endovenous techniques not requiring local anesthesia were relying on sclerotherapy, in one form or another. Particularly, ultrasound guided foam sclerotherapy has achieved widespread popularity because of its perceived low cost and its high availability. Acting as a chemical irritant, foam sclerotherapy is useful for the treatment of the entire spectrum of CEAP class 1 - 6 disease and can be performed using low cost disposables under ultrasound control. However, patients frequently need to return for re-interventions to finally obtain closure of larger veins, repetitively undergoing the risk of specific side effects. These side effects include post-procedure inflammation and long lasting hyperpigmentation of the adjacent skin which is found more frequently than with any other endovenous ablation technology. Moreover, rare but serious side effects like visual disturbances upon injection of the sclerosing agent occur in up to 1.5% of cases[7-9] and stroke related to paradoxical air embolism, although anecdotal, can also occur[10-12].

More recently, a device using mechanical irritation of the endothelium in addition to sclerotherapy was introduced as MechanoChemical Ablation (MOCA)[13]. However, side effects of the MOCA technology may resemble those of sclerotherapy alone, as the dominating mechanism of action still seems to be chemical. Additionally, due to approval related dose limits of the maximum injectable amount of sclerosant, using MOCA, only one great saphenous vein (GSV) can be treated per 24hr period and post-procedural compression is still standard care.

At this point a new endovenous embolisation procedure using a proprietary formulation of CA adhesive has been developed to overcome some of the aforementioned limitations. CA is approved as an implantable medical device in the U.S. for the treatment of arteriovenous malformations and intracranial arterial aneurysms[14], as well as some other indications. Upon intravenous injection of the high-viscosity liquid, CA rapidly polymerizes within seconds and chemically bonds to the inner vein surface eliciting a relatively "cool" inflammatory response, a foreign-body reaction, causing durable occlusion and finally degradation of the implant and the vein.[15-17]

Method
Application System
The disposable VenaSeal Closure System (VCS) currently includes 4 cc of Cyanoacrylate Adhesive and a Delivery System (DS)(Figure 1A). This consists of a 7-F introducer sheath/dilator, a 5-F delivery

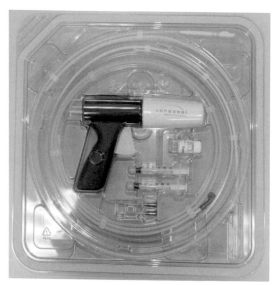

Figure 1: A. Delivery System Kit

catheter, 2x 3ml syringes and dispenser gun. The 5-F delivery catheter has a hydrophobic design to help prevent CA adhesion to the vein wall and a novel configuration with air-filled micro-channels to enhance sonographic visibility (Figure 1B,C). Based on mathematical volumetric calculations in cylindrical systems (venous tubes), engineers designed the dispenser gun to deliver either 0.08 or 0.16 ml of CA with each trigger pull, originally. Later the delivery volume was set to 0.10 ml which is currently still in use.

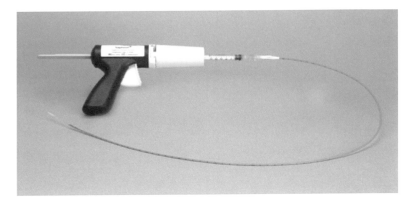

Figure 1: B. mounted components: 7F sheath (blue), housing 5F delivery catheter seen protruding from distal end (clear), attached proximally to dispenser gun.

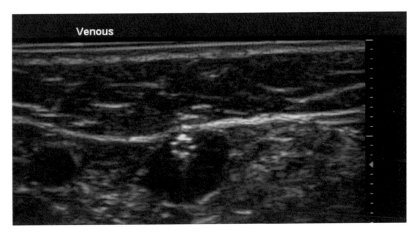

Figure1: C. Ultrasound transverse image sectioning the intravenously placed delivery catheter tip with air channels

Endovenous Placement of the CA-Delivery Catheter

Before the start of CA-treatment, similar to endothermal ablation procedures, the patient's leg veins are mapped under ultrasound guidance to assess the diseased parts of the vein showing pathological reflux. The GSV is then accessed percutaneously at the most distal point of reflux with a micropuncture introducer kit followed by the insertion of a 0.035" J, 180 cm long guide wire. Before the first puncture, a small amount of local anesthesia, approximately 0.5 to 1.0 ml, is injected to minimize discomfort for the patient. No further anesthesia is required and unlike thermal ablation, it is not required along the GSV which is subject to treatment by CA-adhesive embolization.

Using an ultrasound linear scanner in the range of 8-12 MHz, a 7-F introducer sheath/dilator is advanced to the saphenofemoral junction (SFJ) and positioned 5.0 cm caudal to the SFJ. The CA-adhesive and delivery catheter are then prepared. The CA-adhesive is extracted into a 3 ml syringe using a 14G dispenser tip and the syringe is attached to the delivery catheter to fill the tubing

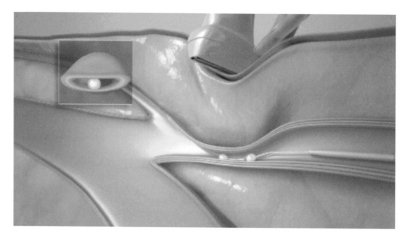

Figure 2: A. A schematic drawing of the placement of the CA-adhesive delivery catheter, sheath and CA-adhesive boluses with respect to the SFJ.

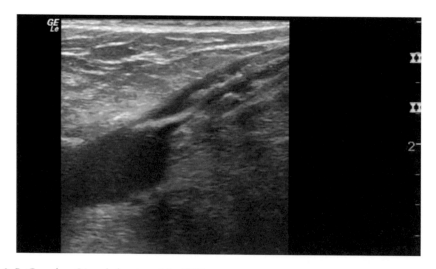

Figure 2: B. Complete CA-embolization of the GSV.

completely up to a laser mark 3cm from the distal tip. The empty delivery catheter tip guarantees prevention of premature contact of CA with blood upon venous insertion and no contact of adhesive within the 7-F introducer sheath. The primed delivery catheter is then inserted into the introducer sheath and secured with a spin-lock mechanism, exposing 5 cm of the delivery catheter tip distal to the end of the sheath. Currently, a distance of 5 cm distal to the SFJ is recommended for catheter placement, which is achieved during catheter insertion, (Figure 2) to avoid glue extensions into the deep vein system. Such glue extensions have been observed in some cases of the first-human-use feasibility study[18] when the distance by protocol was 3-4 cm. To minimize this occurrence, ultrasound guidance is critical during this stage to assure positioning of the catheter in the saphenous vein.

Endovenous Delivery of the CA-Adhesive

The technique of CA-adhesive delivery basically consists of injection of one 0.10ml droplet by pulling and holding the trigger of the dispenser gun for 3 seconds and a subsequent 3 cm pullback of the delivery catheter under moderate external compression exerted by the ultrasound probe and the practitioner's hand. A 30 second polymerization waiting time is required before delivery of the next CA-adhesive droplet. However, the delivery protocol of the initial CA-adhesive delivery 5cm distal to the SFJ varies from this standard - after delivery of the first CA-adhesive droplet the delivery catheter is pulled back 1 cm immediately thereafter followed by injection of another glue droplet. In this

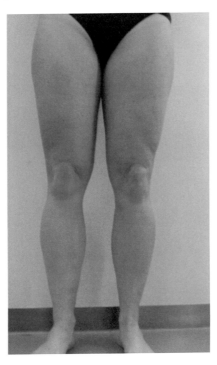

Figure 3: A. Aspect of a patient 24h after CA-adhesive embolization of the right GSV.

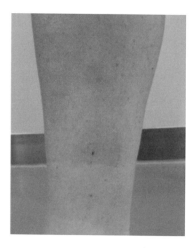

Figure 3: B. detailed view of the puncture site

position a polymerization waiting time of 3 minutes is allowed to pass before CA-adhesive delivery is continued as described above. It must be noted that after glue is dispensed, the catheter must be withdrawn immediately by the required length before polymerisation time is started, to avoid gluing the catheter tip to the vein wall.

Prior to the start of delivery of the CA adhesive, standard instructions for use recommend that the ultrasound transducer is positioned transversely just cephalad to the catheter tip near the SFJ. Once positioned, pressure is applied on the transducer to compress and close the vein 3-4 cm caudal to the SFJ during injection of the first droplet of glue. This injection/retraction process is repeated until the entire length of the target vein segment is treated. The last CA injection is applied approximately 5 cm cephalad to the puncture site. Alternatively, with high quality ultrasound systems axial orientation of the ultrasound probe seems to allow even better control over placement and polymerization of the CA injections and therefore is preferred by the author.

After the catheter is removed, compression is applied to catheter entry site until hemostasis is achieved. A small strip or wound dressing is applied to the puncture site; compression stockings are not required. Twenty four hours post treatment with VenaSeal CA-adhesive, any visible traces of the treatment are rare (Figure 3 A,B).

After treatment the subjects are discharged and instructed to resume normal activities, avoiding strenuous exercise, until the first follow-up visit (24 – 72 hours). No ancillary procedures such as phlebectomy or sclerotherapy are recommended at this time, because they would either require the injection of tumescent local anesthesia or the subsequent use of compression stockings, diluting the pure and minimally invasive character of the CA-adhesive embolization procedure itself.

Results

Up until the time of writing this chapter, animal experiments as well as clinical studies and commercial routine treatments have been performed.

Animal Studies

This comprehensive program, involving 51 animals in total, evaluated the CA material for its intended use at the acute, sub-chronic and chronic time periods. The product tested in these studies is representative of the product used as of this writing. The pre-clinical studies have been conducted in goat, swine and rabbit models to validate the safety and performance of the product, studying:

(1) accuracy of the VenaSeal Adhesive application procedure

(2) ability of acute & chronic vessel closure

(3) acute & chronic toxicity of the implanted adhesive

(4) that the System had an acceptable safety profile and met performance expectations when used as intended.

(5) the Delivery System cannot be accidentally glued to the vessel wall;

(6) the CA can close the vessels in a permanent manner;

(7) that the CA does not migrate from its implant location;

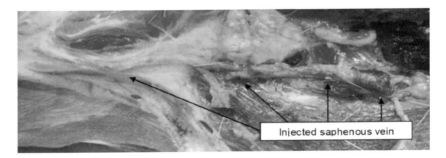

Figure 4: A. Microscopic view of a CA-embolized swine epigastric vein after explantation.

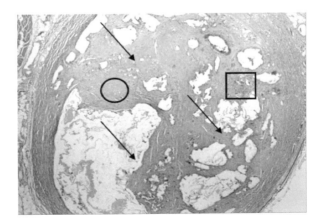

Figure 4: B. Corresponding histopathology after explantation at 30days after treatment showing a foreign body reaction.

- Arrows- Areas of fibrotic cell growth extending into the vein lumen
- Box- Areas of dense fibrosis
- Circle- loose fibrosis present

Each study met the established acceptance criteria, demonstrating that the device operates as intended.

In a swine model, at 30 days[19] after catheter-directed endovenous placement of droplets of 0.16 ml of CA-adhesive every 3 cm in superficial epigastric veins, a granulomatous foreign body reaction was observed in the vein lumen. At 60 days[20], also in swine, fibroblasts were seen invading the contents of the vein lumen and 100% occlusion was observed (Figure 4).

First study in humans - Single Centre Clinical Cohort Study
The first human clinical study was started in December 2010 by treating 8 GSVs in 8 patients. Enrolment was closed in July 2011 after a total of 38 GSVs in 38 patients underwent successful treatment. The study itself was designed as a single-centre, prospective, non-randomized study of feasibility, safety and efficacy in the treatment of GSV incompetence using the VenaSeal CA-adhesive. At baseline, patients were scored using VCSS and CEAP. This was repeated at 48 hours, 1, 3, 6, 12 and 24 months following treatment. Clinical outcomes were assessed with physical examination and duplex ultrasound. Treatment success was defined as complete occlusion of the treated vein segment using duplex ultrasound. Any subject showing patency or recanalization, with or without reflux, in any treated segment greater than 5 cm in length, was considered a failure.

Interestingly, the mean total volume of endovenous CA delivered was only 1.26 +/- 0.44 ml, with a range from 0.63 - 2.25 ml. Immediately after study treatment and at 48h follow-up, 100% of cases demonstrated complete closure of the GSV. One complete and two partial recanalizations were observed during follow-up at 1, 3 and 6 months respectively. Kaplan-Meier analysis yielded an occlusion rate of 92% at 12 months follow-up. Side effects were generally mild and self-limited. The most frequently noted side-effect was phlebitis which was observed in 6 cases (15.8%), requiring NSAIDs for an average period of 5.7 days. Remarkably, in this first human study, eight patients (21.1%) showed thread-like thrombus extensions into the common femoral vein of a mean length of 12.6 mm (range 3.5 – 35 mm) which all resolved spontaneously without clinical sequelae. The VCSS improved in all patients from a mean of 6.1 +/- 2.7 at baseline to 1.1+/-1.0 at 6 months, (p < .0001). Edema improved in 89% of legs (n=34) at 48h follow-up. At 6 months follow-up and without additional adjunctive treatment, 47% of legs (n=17) were free from visible varicosities and an additional 36% (n=13 legs) showed only limited varicosities. The results of this study including the one year follow-up was published in April 2013[18].

European multicentre cohort study
From December 2011 to July 2012 a total of 70 patients were enrolled in a prospective multicentre cohort study in Europe treating 70 incompetent GSVs with VenaSeal CA-adhesive embolization. A one-year preliminary analysis was presented to the 2013 UIP conference in Boston. Seven centres from Germany, UK, Denmark and the Netherlands contributed. Clinical and Duplex follow-up was performed at 48 hours and at 1, 3, 6 and 12 months. The primary endpoint was duplex ultrasound proven GSV closure with lack of pathological reflux at 6 months after study treatment. Inclusion and

Inclusion Criteria

- age ≥18 years and ≤ 70 years
- symptomatic primary GSV incompetence diagnosed by clinical symptoms, with or without visible varicosities, and confirmed by duplex ultrasound imaging#
- CEAP classification of C2, C3 or C4
- ability to walk unassisted
- ability to attend follow-up visits.
- ability to understand the requirements of the study and to provide written informed consent
- maximum GSV diameter on standing pre-procedure ultrasound between 3 and 10 mm.

Exclusion Criteria

- Life expectancy < 1 year.
- Regular pain medication.
- Anticoagulation including Heparin or Coumadin.
- Previous DVT.
- Previous superficial thrombophlebitis in GSV.
- Previous venous treatment on target limb.
- Known Hyper-coagulable disorder.
- Conditions which prevent routine vein treatment like: acute disease, immobilization or inability to ambulate or pregnancy.
- Tortuous GSV, which in the opinion of the Investigator will limit catheter placement. (no 2nd primary access site allowed).
- Incompetent ipsilateral small saphenous or anterior accessory great saphenous vein.
- Known sensitivity to the cyanoacrylate (CA) adhesive.
- Current participation in another clinical study involving an investigational agent or treatment, or within the 30 days prior to enrollment.

Table 1: Inclusion and exclusion criteria of the European multicenter cohort study

exclusion criteria are listed in table 1.

Patients´ characteristics and procedural data were as follows: median age was 48 years [range 22 - 72], median BMI 26.0 [range 18.9-39.0] and median maximum GSV diameter was 8.0 mm [range 2.5 – 14]. CEAP classification stage at baseline was C2 in 29 limbs (41.4%), C3 in 33 limbs (47.1%) and C4 in 8 limbs (11.4%). The median length of the embolized GSV was 38 cm [range 7-72], the median volume of CA delivered was 1.26 ml [range 0.36 - 2.16] corresponding to median number of n = 14 injections [range 4 - 24]. Immediately after study treatment and at 48h follow-up as determined by Duplex ultrasound examination at 48h, all 70 patients (100%) demonstrated anatomical success with fully occluded GSVs without detectable flow or reflux. Additional results cannot be described here before publication in a peer-reviewed Journal.

FDA-IDE trial

Between March and September 2013, 242 patients with 242 incompetent GSVs were enrolled in a FDA-IDE trial which was designed as a United States prospective, randomized control multicentre trial of Cyanoacrylate versus ClosureFast RF-segmental thermal ablation as the control group. In general, this non-inferiority study proved equal results between both study arms in terms of anatomical success. Occlusion rates of the GSV 12 months after the intervention were 97.2% for cyanoacrylate and 97.0% for RF-segmental ablation. More detailed results have been published just recently[21].

Conclusion

Treatment of incompetent GSVs by VenaSeal CA-adhesive embolisation is feasible and safe. Due to the lack of use of anaesthesia except the one injection at the puncture site, the lack of post-interventional compression treatment and a zero-chance for treatment related damage of sensory nerves, it is this author's view that this treatment is by far the least invasive treatment for incompetent saphenous veins to date.

References

1.   Gloviczki P, Comerota AJ, Dalsing MC, Eklof BG, Gillespie DL, Gloviczki ML, Lohr JM, McLafferty RB, Meissner MH, Murad MH, Padberg FT, Pappas PJ, Passman MA, Raffetto JD, Vasquez MA, Wakefield TW; Society for Vascular Surgery; American Venous Forum. The care of patients with varicose veins and associated chronic venous diseases: clinical practice guidelines of the Society for Vascular Surgery and the American Venous Forum. J Vasc Surg. 2011;53(5 Suppl):2S-48S.

2.   Proebstle TM, Gül D, Kargl A, Knop J. Non-Occlusion and early reopening of the great saphenous vein after endovenous laser treatment is fluence dependent. Dermatol Surg. 2004; 30:174-8.

3.   van den Bos R, Arendis L, Kockaert M, et al. Endovenous therapies of lower extremity varicosities: a meta-analysis. J Vasc Surg. 2009;49(1):230-9.

4.   Rasmussen LH, Lawaetz M, Bjoern L, Vennits B, Blemings A, Eklof B. Randomized clinical trial comparing endovenous laser ablation, radiofrequency ablation, foam sclerotherapy and surgical stripping for great saphenous varicose veins. Br J Surg. 2011 Aug;98(8):1079-87.

5.   Almeida JI, Kaufmann J, Gockeritz O, et al. Radiofrequency Endovenous ClosureFAST versus Laser Ablation for the Treatment of Great Saphenous Vein Reflux: A Multicenter, Single-blinded, Randomized Study (RECOVERY Study). J Vasc Interv Radiol. 2009;

20:752-759.

6. Proebstle TM, Vago B, Alm J, Gockeritz O, Lebard C, Pichot O. Treatment of the incompetent great saphenous vein by endovenous radiofrequency powered segmental thermal ablation: First clinical experience. J Vasc Surg. 2008; 47:151-156.

7. Guex JJ, Allaert FA, Gillet JL, Chleir F. Immediate and midterm complications of sclerotherapy: Report of a prospective multicenter registry of 12,173 sclerotherapy sessions. Dermatol Surg. 2005;31:123 – 8

8. Jia X, Mowatt G, Burr JM, Cassar K, Cook J, Fraser C.Systematic review of foam sclerotherapy for varicose veins. Brit J Surg. 2007;94:925 – 36

9. Gillet JL, Guedes JM, Guex JJ, et al. Side effects and com- plications of foam sclerotherapy of the great and small saphenous veins: a controlled multicentre prospective study including 1025 patients. Phlebology. 2009;34:131

10. Forlee MV, Grouden M, Moore DJ, Shanik G. Stroke after varicose vein foam injection sclerotherapy. J Vasc Surg. 2006;43:162 – 4

11. Bush RG, Derrick M, Manjoney D. Major neurological events following foam sclerotherapy. Phlebology. 2008; 23:189 – 92

12. Ma RWL, Pilotelle A, Paraskevas P, Parsi K. Three cases of stroke following peripheral venous interventions. Phlebology. 2011;26:280 – 4

13. Elias S, Raines JK. Mechanochemical tumescentless endovenous ablation: final results of the initial clinical trial. Phlebology. 2012; 27:67-72.

14. Linfante I, Wakhloo AK. Brain aneurysms and arteriovenous malformations: advancements and emerging treatments in endovascular embolization. Stroke. 2007 Apr;38(4):1411-7.

15. Levrier O, Mekkaoui C, Rolland PH, et al. Efficacy and low vascular toxicity of embolization with radical versus anionic polymerization of n-butyl-2-cyanoacrylate (NBCA): An experimental study in the swine. J Neuroradiol. 2003; 30:95-102.

16. Vinters HV, Galil KA, Lundie MJ, Kaufmann JC. The histotoxicity of cyanoacrylates: a selective review. Neuroradiol. 1985; 27:279-291.

17. Spiegel SM, Vinuela F, Goldwasser JM, Fox AJ, Pelz DM. Adjusting the polymerization time of isobutyl-2 cyanoacrylate. Am J Neuroradiol. 1986; 7:109-112.

18. Almeida JI,. Javier JJ, Mackay E, Bautista C, Proebstle TM. First human use of cyanoacrylate adhesive for treatment of saphenous vein incompetence. J Vasc Surg Venous Lymphat Disord. 2013;1:174-80.

19. Min RJ, Almeida JI, McLean DJ, Madsen M, Raabe R. Novel vein closure procedure using a proprietary cyanoacrylate adhesive: 30 swine model results. Phlebology. 2012. Epub 2012 Jan 19.

20. Almeida JI, Min RJ, Raabe R, McLean DJ, Madsen M. Cyanoacrylate adhesive for the closure of truncal veins: 60-day swine model results. Vasc Endovascular Surg. 2011 Oct;45(7):631-5.

21. Morrison N, Gibson K, Vasquez M, Weiss R, Cher D, Madsen M, Jones A.VeClose trial

12-month outcomes of cyanoacrylate closure versus radiofrequency ablation for incompetent great saphenous veins. J Vasc Surg Venous Lymphat Disord. 2017 5:321-330.

Chapter 12

The Changing Face of Ambulatory Venous Surgery in Primary and Recurrent Varicose Veins; Reducing the Number of Therapeutic Visits

Author(s)
Charlotte A Thomas[1,2]
Mark S Whiteley[1,3]

Institution(s)
(1) The Whiteley Clinic, Stirling House, Stirling Road, Guildford, Surrey GU2 7RF
(2) School of Medicine, University of Southampton, UK
(3) Faculty of Health and Biomedical Sciences, University of Surrey, Guildford, Surrey GU2 7XH

Introduction

In recent years, endovenous surgery has become the clear choice in the treatment of varicose veins. Endovenous surgery has shown to be at least as successful as traditional open surgery in many studies[1-4] and is also now the first line treatment for varicose veins in the most recent NICE guidelines[5].

Due to their relatively recent introduction, endovenous techniques only have short term effectiveness data, however they bring many benefits. Patients have less pain, shorter duration of disability, fewer complications, faster return to work and normal activities and a better quality of life[1,3,4,6-10]. There is also evidence emerging that long term recurrence rates with endovenous procedures are low, a 10 year follow up of radiofrequency ablation (RFA) procedures in our unit had a successful closure rate of 96.3%[11].Recurrence rates with traditional surgery are high[7,12]. It is clear that people now understand the advantages of endovenous surgery; the next question is how should endovenous surgery be performed?

The first choice a doctor has regarding endovenous surgery is whether to perform the procedure under a general or local anaesthetic. Both of these have advantages and disadvantages. The advantage of general anaesthetic is that the surgeon can treat all the venous incompetence in one procedure as there are no issues with patient compliance and total dose of local anaesthetic.

In contrast, local anaesthetic has many more advantages. It allows patient feedback directly to the surgeon, reducing the risk of burns during thermoablation or nerve damage during thermoablation or avulsion phlebectomy. A local anaesthetic approach means the patient can eat and drink before the operation which is advantageous especially for diabetics. The combination of being normally hydrated, able to move the legs during the procedure and being ambulatory immediately after the procedure, should decrease the patient's risk of developing a deep vein thrombosis (DVT). Even under general anaesthetic, DVT's have been shown to occur less frequently following endovenous surgery. After RFA, 0.7% of patients develop a DVT and 1% after EVLA[13], compared to open venous surgery where DVT's were found to occur in 5% of patients after the operation[14]. The use of local anaesthetic should also reduce cost. No anaesthetist is required and there is no need for a fully equipped theatre and anaesthetic room, or a bed in a recovery room after the operation.

We began performing endovenous techniques to treat varicose veins under general anaesthetic in 1999 and moved to a local anaesthetic technique in 2005, due to the advantages highlighted above. When using local anaesthetic, a doctor has the option to divide treatment into several sessions, decided by the maximum safe dose of local anaesthetic a patient can be given at one session and also patient compliance with the length of time that it is acceptable to be lying on the operating table.

When endovenous thermoablation first started under local anaesthetic using tumescence in the United States, it was common to treat only one truncal vein per session. The amount of work that can be performed in one session during vein surgery is still a hot topic of discussion in the vein world. The Ambulatory Varicosity avUlsion Later or Synchronised (AVULS) study is, at the time of writing this chapter, currently researching into whether RFA with concomitant phlebectomy compared to sequential phlebectomy or foam sclerotherapy will result in an improvement in disease specific quality of life at 6 months, will reduce the need for further procedures and will be more cost effective[15].

A separate study has already been found that EVLA with concomitant phlebectomy reduced the need for secondary procedures and significantly improved quality of life and severity of venous disease[16]. Conversely, there is also a feeling that delaying other treatment such as phlebectomies or foam sclerotherapy after initial truncal vein closure may result in less treatment being needed overall, due to smaller tributary veins reducing in diameter as a result of truncal vein ablation.

With our extensive experience in performing endovenous surgery, we decided to analyse the evolution of local anaesthetic endovenous treatment in our own clinic between 2006 and 2011. By 2006 we already had 7 years of experience in endovenous techniques at the clinic, although at that stage, most of our treatments had been under general anaesthetic. As such our doctors were highly competent in the endovenous techniques such as EVLA, RFA and trans-luminal occlusion of perforators (TRLOP).

In 2005, when we had initially decided to change from using general anaesthetic to treating varicose veins under local anaesthetic as ambulatory procedures in the clinic, we surveyed what seemed to be standard practice throughout the world at that time, amongst the few clinics performing such surgery. Following what appeared to be the usual practice in such units at that time, we decided to treat individual truncal veins in separate visits to the clinic.

However, with increasing experience of the local anaesthetic approach, we found that we were able to treat increasingly more incompetent truncal veins within a safe dose of local anaesthetic and within patient tolerance. This allowed us to treat more truncal veins per session, reducing the number of endovenous devices used per patient and number of sessions each patient required to treat all of their venous incompetence. Although there was a clear change in our practice, which evolved with experience, we felt it was important to quantify this change by investigating the progression of our endovenous techniques between 2006 and 2011.

Method

We took a "snapshot" sample of patients from the same month each year between 2006 and 2011 for comparison. Patients undergoing any procedure for venous incompetence at the clinic during October in each year were included. A session was classified as a single appointment at the clinic where the patient has one or more of the following treatments performed: EVLA, RFA, TRLOP, phlebectomy or foam sclerotherapy.

A retrospective review of all patient notes and theatre records was performed. Patient demographics including age, sex and parity if female was noted for each patient. The number of procedures, endovenous devices used and reflux patterns were also recorded for every patient in the study. To ensure that our patients were similar in each year of the study, statistical tests were performed to check for any significant differences between the patient groups.

Results

Two hundred and ninety six patients were included in the study and a breakdown of patient demographics can be seen in Table 1.

The extent of venous disease in each leg was classified according to the CEAP classification, with 366 of 522 legs (70.1%) being classed as CEAP clinical score 2 (C2), with the mode being C2 in each year of the study. It is of note that the number of legs classed as C2 fell between 2009 to 2010, with a simultaneous increase in the number of legs classified as C3 and C4, suggesting that the severity of disease in new patients attending the clinic increased over the study period.

In order to review how our treatment evolved over the six years the population studied must be similar, so we performed statistical tests to identify any differences between the annual groups. An ANOVA statistical analysis was performed to compare patient age between all the years of the study and this found a statistically significant difference (P=0.034) although there was no discernable trend

	Number of patients	Number of legs treated	Patient age			M/F ratio			P/R legs			1 or 2 legs treated		
			Mean	Low	High	M	F	F (%)	P	R	P (%)	1 leg	2 legs	2 legs (%)
2006	28	53	55.7	31	78	6	22	78.57	40	13	75.5	3	25	89.3
2007	52	86	48.8	25	70	12	40	76.92	59	27	68.6	18	34	65.4
2008	51	88	53.4	36	89	7	44	86.27	51	37	58.0	14	37	72.6
2009	53	95	52.4	26	72	6	47	88.68	67	28	70.5	11	42	79.3
2010	48	85	56.3	32	82	10	38	79.17	52	33	61.2	11	37	77.1
2011	64	115	52.1	28	85	11	53	82.81	63	52	54.8	13	51	79.7

Table 1. A breakdown of patient demographics by year. (M = Male; F = Female; P = primary venous reflux; R = recurrent venous reflux)

throughout the study period. Chi-squared tests were performed to compare the male to female ratio of each year, the ratio of primary and recurrent incompetence in each year and the ratio of whether the patient had bilateral or unilateral treatment. No statistically significant difference (P>0.05) was found between any of the years in any of these variables.

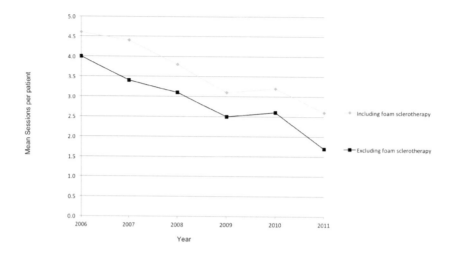

Figure 1: Graph showing the mean number of sessions per patient for each year between 2006 and 2011. All treatment sessions including foam sclerotherapy are shown in grey and treatment sessions excluding foam sclerotherapy only are shown in black.

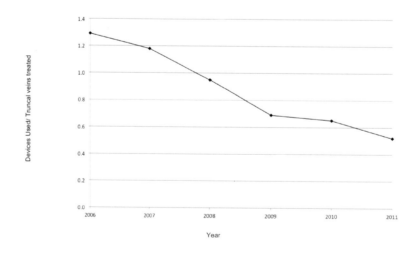

Figure 2: Graph showing the number of endovenous devices used divided by the number of truncal veins treated, for each year between 2006 and 2011.

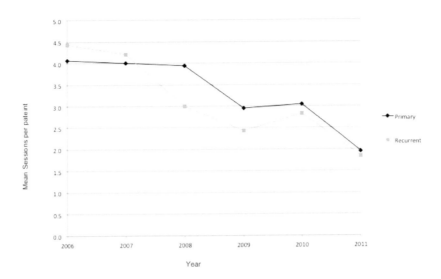

Figure 3: Graph showing the mean number of total treatment sessions (including foam sclerotherapy) per patient for the treatment of primary varicose veins (black line) and the treatment of recurrent varicose veins (grey line), between 2006 and 2011.

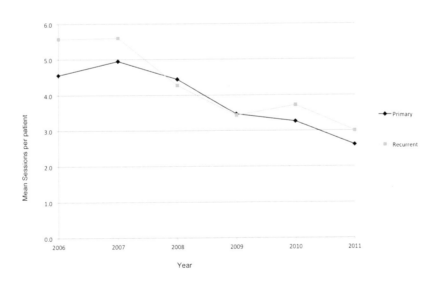

Figure 4: Graph showing the mean number of treatment sessions (excluding foam sclerotherapy) per patient for the treatment of primary varicose veins (black line) and the treatment of recurrent varicose veins (grey line), between 2006 and 2011.

Despite not being statistically significant, it is noteworthy that the ratio of primary varicose veins is higher in 2006 and 2009, at 40 of 53 legs (75.5%) and 67 of 95 legs (70.5%) respectively, whereas in 2011 this was lower at 63 of 115 legs (54.8%). This shows that during the study period there was a tendency to more patients being treated with recurrent varicose veins. All differences were taken into consideration while analysing the results.

We found that between 2006 and 2011 the number of sessions and endovenous devices used per patient considerably decreased. The mean number of sessions per patient, excluding foam sclerotherapy, decreased every year except for 2010 (Fig.1) and the difference between 2006 and 2011 was statistically significant (Mann-Whitney U Test U=1573.5 P=2x10-6).

The mean number of endovenous devices used per patient decreased every year from 2.7 endovenous devices in 2006 to 1.2 endovenous devices in 2011. When taking into account how many incompetent truncal veins were treated, this number also decreased every year (Fig. 2). The difference in the number of endovenous devices used per truncal vein treated from 2006 to 2011 is statistically significant (Mann-Whitney U Test U=1603.5 P=2x10-6).

We also found a difference in the number of procedures and endovenous devices needed to treat primary or recurrent varicose veins. Patients with primary varicose veins required on average more procedures, excluding foam sclerotherapy, than patients with recurrent incompetence. Over the study period, the mean number of procedures for primary varicose veins was 3.2 per patient and for recurrent varicose veins it was 2.8 per patient, this was statistically significant (Mann-Whitney U test U=7403 P=0.024) (Fig. 3). When we included foam sclerotherapy, the mean number of procedures for primary incompetence was 3.8 procedures per patient compared to recurrent incompetence which had a mean of 4.0 procedures per patient (not statistically significant) (Fig. 4).

Discussion

This study shows that despite a fairly consistent population, the number of procedures each patient undergoes and the number of endovenous devices used per patient has decreased between 2006 and 2011. This outcome is advantageous for both the patients and the funders of healthcare. This decreasing pattern was the same for all the subgroups of patients, whether they had primary or recurrent reflux and whether they had bilateral or unilateral treatment.

These reductions demonstrate our increasing experience in local anaesthetic treatment of varicose veins. In the early years of local anaesthetic endovenous surgery, it was perceived 'standard practice' to treat one truncal vein per session. However, with experience, we found we were able to treat more incompetent truncal veins per session, whilst keeping within patient tolerance and the maximum safe dose of local anaesthetic.

At first look it may appear surprising that more than one endovenous device was used per incompetent truncal vein as one might expect that the most endovenous devices we could use for one truncal vein would be one endovenous device. However it has always been our practice to treat incompetent perforating veins (IPV) with TRLOP using endovenous devices[17]. More than one endovenous device was commonly required per patient because they were treated over a number of visits to the clinic and so a new device had to be used each time, as was common practice in most ambulatory vein clinics in 2006. By 2011 we were using a mean of just 0.5 endovenous devices per incompetent truncal vein treated. This low result is due to the fact that we were able to treat several incompetent truncal veins in one treatment episode and also use the same endovenous device for treating IPV's with TRLOP wherever possible.

The ANOVA statistical test found that patient age in each year group was statistically significantly different. However, for the purpose of this study, small differences in age will have had little impact on the considerable decrease in the number of procedures and endovenous devices needed to treat each patient. In addition, there was no trend in the age differences over the study period.

Between 2009 and 2010 there was a small but consistent increase in the number of sessions each patient had, excluding foam sclerotherapy. This rise was seen in patients who had had treatment for primary or recurrent varicose veins in both legs. Looking at the patient demographics, in 2010 the mean patient age was marginally higher than other years at 56.3 years. Between 2009 and 2010 the severity of venous reflux disease increased; the percentage of legs with a CEAP clinical score of C2 decreased and the number of legs scoring C3 and C4 increased. Hence, the increased severity of venous reflux disease may have increased the number of procedures each patient required to have their reflux treated successfully. However, as the increase was marginal, it is only noticeable as it bucks the trend of a steady decrease. Therefore, it is likely that this reflects that we were working to a protocol, using the techniques available in those years, whilst continuing to evolve our technique.

It is interesting that there is a great similarity in the number of sessions required for patients with primary incompetence and patients with recurrent incompetence. Looking at the number of sessions per patient excluding treatment with foam sclerotherapy, fewer sessions were needed on the patients with recurrent varicose veins. One explanation for this could be that recurrent veins are more difficult to treat with endovenous techniques and are often treated with phlebectomies and foam sclerotherapy alone. With this in mind, we looked at the number of sessions per patient including treatment with foam sclerotherapy and found that the mean number of sessions on patients with primary incompetence is slightly lower than those with recurrent incompetence at 3.9 sessions and 4.0 respectively.

This suggests that on average, patients with recurrent reflux need fewer endovenous procedures, but more foam sclerotherapy than patients with primary varicose veins so overall there is no difference in the number of sessions required.

There was an increase in the number of patients with recurrent disease over the study period. This is due to an increase in the number of patients with recurrent varicose veins being referred to our unit, having been previously treated elsewhere.

This study shows the development of what is possible with regards to the endovenous treatment of incompetent superficial leg veins. With current technology we feel we are at the limit for the fewest number of sessions and endovenous devices each patient requires to have their venous incompetence treated fully. Fewer visits are advantageous to the patient and the use of fewer sessions and devices will reduce the cost to the funders of healthcare. We are now at a stage where we are able to treat more venous incompetence per session without compromising our high quality of treatment and success rates, shown by our internal audits and our patient satisfaction[18].

Although the results of this study does not allow us to predict the number of endovenous devices and procedures for each patient individually, it does help us to predict the number of procedures and endovenous devices that a group of patients are likely to require to treat their venous reflux and allows us to plan appropriate resources. It may also be useful for funders of healthcare to use such data when planning resources that will be required for patients with varicose veins or venous reflux (see Table 2 for predicted figures).

	Mean total procedures	Mean procedures excluding foam sclerotherapy	Mean number of endovenous devices needed per patient
Bilateral treatment for primary venous reflux	2.6	2.0	1.4
Bilateral treatment for recurrent venous reflux	3.0	1.9	1.3
Unilateral treatment for primary venous reflux	1.6	1.0	0.9

Table 2. Predictions of future needs based on our 2011 results.

Conclusions

Endovenous surgery has revolutionised venous treatments over the last decade and a half. As with all new medical advances, the early research was aimed at developing the techniques themselves and checking the success rates of all of the new procedures. As endovenous surgery is now becoming widely accepted to be the optimal treatment for varicose veins and venous reflux disease, it has now become necessary to show the optimal way of delivering the treatment.

Our 14 year experience has helped shape our protocols and this study, looking at the development of our endovenous practice under local anaesthesia between 2006 and 2011, has shown some interesting developments. Firstly, we were able to see a change from the widely accepted one visit and one procedure per truncal vein needing treatment in 2006, to multiple veins being treated at each session by 2011. In addition, we were able to note a decrease in the total number of sessions as well as the total number of devices required to treat patients.

Looking at both primary and recurrent varicose veins, we found an interesting result in that, contrary to what might be thought, patients with recurrent varicose veins require fewer endovenous devices on average than those with primary varicose veins. However this is balanced by an increase in the number of foam sclerotherapy sessions required in patients with recurrent varicose veins when compared to patients with primary varicose veins.

These results will help decrease the costs and resource implications of endovenous surgery under local anaesthesia whilst maintaining clinical results.

References

1. Nesbitt C, Eifell RKG, Coyne P, Badri H, Bhattacharya V, Stansby G. Endovenous ablation (radiofrequency and laser) and foam sclerotherapy versus conventional surgery for great saphenous vein varices. Cochrane Database of Systematic Reviews 2011;(10):CD005624. DOI: 10.1002/14651858.CD005624.pub2

2. Dindyal S, Woddburn KR. Changing practice from conventional surgery to endovenous treatments produces excellent results for both long and short saphenous varicose veins. Ann R Coll Surg Engl. 2010;92:85-90

3. Hinchcliffe RJ, Ubhi J, Beech A, Ellison J, Braithwaite BD. A Prospective Randomised Controlled Trial of VNUS Closure versus Surgery for the Treatment of Recurrent Long Saphenous Varicose Veins. Eur J Vasc Endovasc Surg. 2006;31:212-8

4. Min RJ, Khilnani N, Zimmet SE. Endovenous Laser Treatment of Saphenous Vein Reflux: Long-Term Results. JVIR. 2003;14(8):991-6

5. Varicose veins in the legs: The diagnosis and management of varicose veins – CG168 (http://publications.nice.org.uk/varicose-veins-in-the-legs-cg168) (accessed 5 Aug 2013)

6. Murad H, Coto-Yglesias F, Zumaeta-Garcia M et al. A systematic review and meta-analysis of the treatments of varicose veins. J Vasc Surg. 2011;53(165):49S-65S

7. Lurie F, Creton D, Eklof B et al. Prospective Randomised Study of Endovenous Radiofrequency Obliteration (closure) Versus Ligation and Vein Stripping (EVOLVeS): Two-year Follow-up. Eur J Vasc Endovasc Surg. 2005;29:67-73

8. Ugur Ozkan, Sariturk C. Early clinical improvement in chronic venous insufficiency symptoms after laser ablation of saphenous veins. Diagn Interv Radiol. 2012 Jul (ePub ahead of print)

9. Vuylsteke M, Van den Bussche D, Audenaert EA, Lissens P. Endovenous laser obliteration for the treatment of primary varicose veins. Phlebology. 2006;21:80-87.

10. McBride KD. Changing to endovenous treatment for varicose veins: How much more evidence is needed? The Surgeon. 2011;9(3):150-9

11. Taylor D, Whiteley A, Fernandez-Hart T, Whiteley M Ten Year Results of Radiofrequency Ablation (VNUS Closure®) of the Great Saphenous and Anterior Accessory Saphenous Veins in the Treatment of Varicose Veins. Tecnicas endovasculares. April 2013;Vol XVI (1):134

12. Allaf N, Welch M. Recurrent varicose veins: Inadequate surgery remains a problem. Phlebology. 2005;20:138–40

13. Marsh P, Price BA, Holdstock J, Harrison C, Whiteley MS. Deep Vein Thrombosis (DVT) after Venous Thermoablation Techniques: Rates of Endovenous Heat-induced Thrombosis (EHIT) and Classical DVT after Radiofrequency and Endovenous Laser Ablation in a Single Centre. Eur J Vasc Endovasc Surg. 2010;40(4):521-7

14. Van Rij AM, Chai J, Hill GB, Christie RA. Incidence of deep vein thrombosis after varicose vein surgery. Br J Surg. 2004;91:1582-5.

15. UK Clinical trials gateway. Ambulatory Varicosity avUlsion Later or Synchronised (AVULS).

http://www.ukctg.nihr.ac.uk/trialdetails/ISRCTN76821539 (accessed 12 Jul 2013)

16. Carradice D, Mekako AI, Hatfield J, Chetter IC. Randomized clinical trial of concomitant or sequential phlebectomy after endovenous laser therapy for varicose veins. Br J Surg. 2009 Apr;96(4):369-75.

17. Bacon JL, Dinneen AJ, Marsh P, Holdstock JM, Price BA, Whiteley MS. Five-year results of incompetent perforator vein closure using TRans-Luminal Occlusion of Perforator. Phlebology. 2009;24(2):74-8

18. Whiteley MS. Patient Satisfaction. http://www.thewhiteleyclinic.co.uk/patient_satisfaction. htm (accessed 12 Jul 2013)

Chapter 13

Patient Experience of Conscious Surgery

Author(s)
Bryony Hudson[1]
Mark S Whiteley[1,2]

Institution(s)
(1) The Whiteley Clinic, Stirling House, Stirling Road, Guildford, Surrey GU2 7RF
(2) Faculty of Health and Biomedical Sciences, University of Surrey, Guildford, Surrey GU2 7XH

Introduction

As surgery moves away from traditional methods and models of hospital based recovery, qualitative and quantitative research has been conducted to examine how these changes affect the experience of surgical patients. Understanding patients' perspectives and experiences can facilitate the modification and improvement of services and potentially post-operative outcomes such as pain and return to work[1]. This chapter looks at factors that have been identified by patients as anxiety provoking, the impact this anxiety can have on both intra and post-operative outcomes and suggestions for non-pharmacological anxiety and pain management during conscious surgery. The chapter concludes with an overview of how The Whiteley Clinic has responded to the deficit in research in this area.

The relationship between anxiety, pain and post-surgical outcomes

Research has indicated that anxiety is a common response to surgery[2] but the prospect of being conscious during surgery can be fraught with a range of specific fears and anxieties[3,4]. Such stressors include the sounds and sights of the operating theatre[5], the prospect of feeling the surgeon's touch[6] and concerns surrounding anaesthesia[7].

The relationships between psychological factors such as anxiety, the immune system and post-surgical recovery are widely accepted and have considerable implications for conscious surgery practices[8,9]. Not only is anxiety unpleasant, but a consistent relationship has been observed between surgical anxieties, post-operative pain[10,11], increased analgesic requirements[12] and delayed recovery[13]. Furthermore, increased anxiety can reduce pain thresholds[14] and is also implicated in elevated pain intensity estimates[15,16].

So what are the mechanisms behind this relationship? It is known that elevated anxiety triggers both physiological and behavioural responses. These include immune function suppression, hyperactivation of the hypothalamic-pituitary axis[17,18] and importantly for pain perception, an increased focus on threatening stimuli[19]. This focus on threatening, or pain related, stimuli is a consideration in models of pain perception. The level of pain we experience is thought to be influenced by an evaluation of the sensory, affective and cognitive information[20] to which we attend and also information from our previous experiences. Pain perception is therefore influenced by a range of factors cognitive, sensory and affective in nature and the interactions between them. Using cognitive principles to reduce anxiety pre and intra-operatively will not only improve patient's experience but also decrease the risk of adverse reactions after surgery leading to faster, less painful recoveries.

Using distraction for pain and anxiety management in a surgical context

Distraction is a method of cognitive refocusing which shifts attention from painful or anxiety provoking stimuli towards less threatening, more pleasant stimuli. Research into the application of distraction interventions in surgical contexts, while in its infancy, is beginning to emerge which suggests that distraction could be a simple and low cost non-pharmacological adjunct to traditional pain management strategies.

The mechanisms through which distraction is thought to influence our perception of pain relates back to models of pain and attention. As we have limited cognitive capacity we are unable to attend to every stimuli in our environment and as painful or threatening stimuli have the greatest salience, our attention is drawn towards them. The addition of pleasant novel stimuli used in distraction interventions aim to divert our limited cognitive resources away from threatening stimuli towards pleasant, non-threatening stimuli. This shift in attentional focus leaves less cognitive capacity available for pain perception[21]. Psychological factors such as anxiety and mood can also impact upon the type of information to which we attend, particularly in situations such as surgery in which we perceive a lack of control. Therefore, providing an engaging and uplifting distraction has the potential to work on two levels, improving mood and reducing the cognitive capacity available for pain perception.

Various distraction techniques have been hypothesised to be effective in pain and anxiety management and a short summary of some of the most effective distractions now follows:

Music

Music has been found to be efficacious in lowering physiological indicators of anxiety such as heart rate[22], respiratory rate, sweat gland activity, blood pressure and epinephrine levels[23] in a range of medical settings. Additionally, music has been shown to influence pain medication requirements and recovery rates following surgery[24,25]. There are various hypotheses as to why music may be beneficial in a medical context, it could be that music masks sounds of the operating theatre (which have previously been identified as stressors in this context,[5]), or it could be that music induces a state of relaxation which decreases anxiety and perception of pain.

A review of the literature regarding the efficacy of conscious surgery shows encouraging results. Patients who received a musical intervention were found to report lower pain scores during varicose vein surgery than patients who received treatment as usual (TAU) in a randomised controlled trial[26]. Further research[27] demonstrated that the timing of the musical intervention (either during or after surgery) did not significantly impact the benefit it delivered in terms of pain reduction in the first 2 post-operative hours, with both being superior to TAU. While there is currently limited evidence exploring the potential benefits of providing music as a distraction for patients undergoing varicose vein surgery, the efficacy of this distraction in other patient groups has generated support for its use. Further research is warranted into the use of music as a non-pharmacological adjunct to surgery given the benefits observed and the ease with which it can be implemented in surgical settings.

Audio visual distraction techniques

The evidence supporting the use of music suggests audio visual distractions could also be beneficial for surgical patients. According to theories of pain, increasing the amount of distracting, pleasant stimuli the patient experiences should decrease the amount of pain perceived. This was confirmed in a randomised controlled trial conducted in China[28], which was one of the first to investigate the anti-anxiolytic properties of watching a DVD during surgery. Participants in the experimental condition were given a choice of DVD which they watched during their procedure. Anxiety was assessed using the state trait anxiety inventory (STAI) and a visual analogue scale (VAS) in the operating theatre before surgery, 15 minutes after the start of surgery and post-operatively. Compared to the control group, who received usual standard care, participants who watched a DVD reported significantly lower intra-operative anxiety.

To our knowledge, there is currently no published research regarding the impact of audio visual distraction on patient reported anxiety and pain amongst patients receiving varicose vein surgery. The limited evidence available and the ease with which this type of distraction could be implemented in operating theatres suggest that the use of audio visual stimuli is an area in which further research is required.

Touch

Early research into the effects of massage for patients undergoing conscious surgery has proved positive[29]. Patients who received five minutes of pre-operative hand massage reported significantly lower post-operative anxiety than patients who received TAU following cataract surgery under local anaesthetic. In terms of intra-operative anxiety management, Simmons et al.[30] found that participants who received usual care with massage during ocular injections prior to cataract surgery reported significantly less pain and anxiety than patients who received standard care alone.

Reflexology is another form of massage that can be applied to either hands or feet[31]. Chanif, Petpichtchian and Chongchareon[32] reviewed 8 studies investigating the effects of foot reflexology on post-operative pain (5 randomised controlled trials and 3 quasi experimental trials). Seven of the 8 reviewed studies concluded that reflexology resulted in significant reductions in pain or anxiety. This is an impressive result however the authors highlight a number of limitations concerning the quality of the evidence reviewed. Differences in reflexology administration protocols, surgical procedures, analgesic medications and marked differences in baseline scores between control and experimental groups were noted in half of the studies reviewed.

In the light of these promising findings, further robust research is needed to enable firm conclusions to be drawn regarding the potential benefits of touch as a form of distraction for conscious surgery patients.

Current research

This chapter has provided a brief overview of the causes and impact of surgical anxiety and how distraction could be used to counter these effects. In response to the gaps identified in the current literature, the authors of this chapter have completed a large scale multi-method study exploring the efficacy of four distraction interventions (music, audio visual stimuli, touch and interaction) in comparison with TAU on immediate and longer term outcomes following varicose vein surgery[33].

Our results indicate that the addition of simple, affordable intra-operative distraction to minimally invasive surgery for varicose veins can significantly improve patient experience in comparison to TAU. Patient reported intra-operative anxiety ratings were significantly lower in the interaction, touch and DVD conditions compared to controls while significantly lower intra-operative pain ratings (NRS) were observed in the touch and interaction conditions. These results support previous work on the role of distraction in improving patient experience and also reflect the importance of the nurses' role in the operating theatre. Therefore we support their use, or the option of their use in routine practice. Providing intra-operative distraction in the form of nurse-patient interaction, tactile stimulation such as stress balls or audio visual stimulation in the form of a DVD are useful adjuncts to TAU and should be considered as an option for all local anaesthetic surgical procedures.

The authors believe that given the minimal cost and invasiveness of the distraction interventions studied, and the benefits observed in response to their addition to TAU, that patients and health care providers should be aware of these findings to allow them to make informed decisions regarding the management of intra-operative pain and anxiety.

Conclusions

The rise of conscious surgery for varicose veins has a number of implications for health care providers. In hand with the numerous benefits of conscious, day case surgery comes a new set of responsibilities towards patients at all stages of the operative experience, and in particular in the operating theatre. Research has shown that despite appreciating the benefits of conscious surgery, many patients experience a degree of anxiety both before and during their procedure. While research into the methodology and objective outcomes of varicose vein surgery has achieved much in recent years, it appears that research into the psychological impact of these developments has not flourished alongside.

References

1.   Costa MJ. The lived perioperative experience of ambulatory surgery patients. AORN.

2001;74(6), 874-881.

2. Pierangotti P, Covelli G, Vario M. Anxiety, stress and preoperative nursing. Professioni infermieristiche. 2002; 55:180-191

3. Mitchell M. Patient anxiety and modern elective surgery: a literature review. J Clin Nurs. 2003;12(6): 806-815.

4. Wetsch WA, Pircher I, Lederer W, Kinzl JF, Traweger C, Heinz-Erian P, Benzer A. Preoperative stress and anxiety in day-care patients and inpatients undergoing fast-track surgery. Br J Anaes. 2009; 103(2): 199-205.

5. Mitchell M. Conscious surgery: influence of the environment on patient anxiety. J Adv Nurs. 2008; 64(3): 261-271

6. Mitchell M. Patient anxiety and conscious surgery. J Perio Prac. 2009; 19(6): 168-173.

7. Mitchell M. A patient-centred approach to day surgery nursing. Nurs Stand. 2010; 24(44): 40-46

8. O'Leary A. Stress, emotion, and human immune function. Psych Bull. 1990; 108(3): 363

9. Vollmer-Conna U, Bird KD, Yeo BW, Truskett PG, Westbrook RF, Wakefield D. Psychological factors, immune function and recovery from major surgery. Acta Neuropsych. 2009; 21(4): 169-178.

10. Carr EC, Thomas NV, Wilson-Barnet J. Patient experiences of anxiety, depression and acute pain after surgery: a longitudinal perspective. Int J Nurs Stud. 2005; 42(5): 521-530.

11. Ip HYV, Abrishami A, Peng P, Wong J, Chung F. Predictors of postoperative pain and analgesic consumption. Anesthesiology. 2009; 111: 657-77

12. Powell R, Johnston M, Smith WC, King PM, Chambers WA, Krukowski Z. Psychological risk factors for chronic post-surgical pain after inguinal hernia repair surgery: A prospective cohort study. Eur J Pain. 2011; 16 (4): 600-610

13. Mavros MN, Athanasiou S, Gkegkes I D, Olyzos KA, Peppas G, Falagas ME. Do psychological variables affect early surgical recovery? PLOSone. 2011; (6): 5. e20306

14. Rhudy JL, Meagher MW. Fear and anxiety: Divergent effects on human pain thresholds. Pain. 200; 84: 65-75

15. Seidman L, Lung K, Nailboff B, Zelter L, Tsao J. Sensitisation to laboratory pain stimuli in healthy children and adolescents is associated with higher ratings of anxiety, pain intensity and pain bother. J Pain. 2014; 15 (4): 53

16. Kain ZN, Mayes LC, Caldwell-Andrews AA, Karas DE, McClain BC. Preoperative anxiety, postoperative pain, and behavioral recovery in young children undergoing surgery. Pediatrics. 2006; 118 (2): 651-658.

17. Kiecolt-Glaser JK, Page GG, Marucha PT, MacCallum RC, Glaser R. Psychological influences on surgical recovery: Perspectives from psychoneuroimmunology. Am Psychol. 1998; 53(11): 1209-1218.

18. Tsigos C, Chrousos GP. Hypothalamic–pituitary–adrenal axis, neuroendocrine factors and stress. J Psychos Res. 2002; 53(4): 865-871

19.   Bar-Haim Y, Lamy D, Pergamin L, Bakermans-Kranenburg MJ, Van Ijzendoorn MH. Threat related attentional bias in anxious and non anxious individuals: A meta-analytic study. Psycho Bull. 2007; 133(1): 1-24.

20.   Melzack R, Torgerson WS. On the language of pain. Anaesthesiology.1971; 34: 50–59.

21.   Ruscheweyh R, Kreusch A, Albers C, Sommer J,Marziniak M. The effect of distraction strategies on pain perception and the nociceptive flexor reflex (RIII reflex). Pain. 2011;152 (11): 2662-2671

22.   Allen K, Golden LH, Izzo Jr JL, Ching MI, Forrest A, Niles CR, Barlow JC. Normalization of hypertensive responses during ambulatory surgical stress by perioperative music. Psychosom Med. 2001; 63(3): 487-492.

23.   Arslan S, Ozer N, Ozyurt F. Effect of music on preoperative anxiety in men undergoing urogenital surgery. Aus J Advan Nurs. 2001; 26(2): 46.

24.   Sen H, Yanarateş O, Sızlan A, Kılıç E, Ozkan S, Dağli G. The efficiency and duration of the analgesic effects of musical therapy on postoperative pain. J Turk Soc Algology. 2010; 22(4): 145-150.

25.   Nilsson U, Rawal N, Uneståhl LE, Zetterberg C, Unosson M. Improved recovery after music and therapeutic suggestions during general anaesthesia: a double-blind randomised controlled trial. Acta Anaes Scand. 2001; 45(7): 812-817.

26.   Nilsson U, Rawal N, Enqvist B, Unosson M Analgesia following music and therapeutic suggestions in the PACU in ambulatory surgery; a randomized controlled trial. Acta Anaes Scan. 2003; 47(3): 278-283

27.   Nillsson U, Rawal N, Unosson M. A comparison of intra operative or post operative exposure to music—a controlled trial of the effects on postoperative pain. Anaesthesia. 2003; 58(7): 699-703.

28.   Man AKY, Yap JCM.The effect of intraoperative video on patient anxiety. Anaesthesia. 2003; 58 (1): 64-68

29.   Kim MS, Cho KS, Woo HM, Kim JH. Effects of hand massage on anxiety in cataract surgery using local anaesthesia. J Cat Refra Surg. 2001; 27(6): 884-890.

30.   Simmons D, Chabal C, Griffith J, Rausch M, Steele B. A clinical trial of distraction techniques for pain and anxiety control during cataract surgery. Insight. 2004; 29 (4): 13-16

31.   Gunnarsdottir T, Jonsdottir H. Does the experimental design capture the effects of complimentay therapy? A study using reflexology for patients undergoing coronary artery bypass surgery. J Clin Nurs. 2007;16 (4): 777-785

32.   Chanif C, Petpichetchian W, Chongchareon W. Does foot massage relieve acute postoperative pain? A literature review. Nur Med J Nurs. 2013; 3 (1): 483-397

33.   Hudson BF, Davidson J, Whiteley MS. The impact of hand reflexology on pain , anxiety and satisfaction during minimally invasive surgery underlocal anaesthetic: a randomised controlled trial. Int J Nurse Stud. 2015; 52(12): 1989-97.

Chapter 14

Patient Reported Outcomes and Quality of Life Scores in Assessing the success of varicose vein surgery

Author(s)
Tristan R A Lane
Alun H Davies

Institution(s)
Academic Section of Vascular Surgery, Imperial College London and Imperial Healthcare NHS Trust.

Introduction
Varicose veins are extremely common and chronic venous insufficiency has a wide spectrum of disease. Fortunately venous duplex ultrasound provides us with excellent anatomical and haemodynamic detail[1]. Sadly this does not always correlate well with patient symptomatology, the disease process or post-surgical outcomes[2-4]. Patients vary from those with extensive skin changes without symptoms to those with minor symptomatic varicosities. Additionally recurrence and progression of the disease

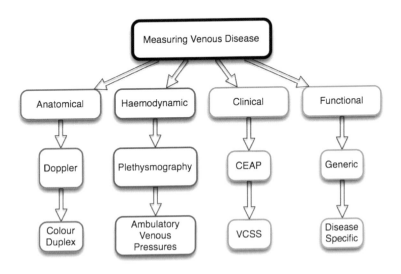

Figure 1: The different methods of measuring venous disease

has led to UK funding bodies rationing treatment based on recurrence rates of 50% at five years[5], which is in conflict with the published evidence[6,7], and the Department of Health's own figures, which for April-December 2012 showed that 97% of patients' symptoms improved, by an average of 38% (calculated from provisional Hospital Episode Statistics).

With this confusion, how does one begin to assess which patients benefit and which do not? How do you assess whether you have successfully treated your patients? Crucially how do you manage their expectations[8] - is complete removal of all visible veins and symptoms actually the patient's expectation, and is this the only true success?

Figure 1 describes the various methods of assessment.

Anatomical

Anatomic data is immensely reassuring to the clinician and the patient if symptoms have improved. A full colour duplex scan of the treated vein will ensure that the treatment is a technical success. However, this is only useful as an adjunct to a clear review of the patient's symptoms, as it will not detect residual swelling, residual varicosities, paraesthesia or skin discolouration. Additionally it requires specialist skills and is time-consuming. The assessment of the post-treatment vein is not straight-forward and requires experience[9,10]. The presence of re-canalisation does not necessarily indicate recurrence and may have no significant effect on venous flow. These scanning complications are mirrored after open surgery[11].

Over the past decade, since the introduction of endovenous treatments, research has moved from this technical aspect towards assessment of patient success as occlusion rates have been found to be broadly similar in the region of 95%, and comparable to surgery[6,7,12].

Finally, if a patient is asymptomatic, then the presence of failed treatment is inconsequential - one would not re-treat the patient. This is of interest from a training and research perspective only.

Haemodynamic

Haemodynamic assessment post-treatment is again very reassuring and provides proof of improved venous outflow. However, this assessment is complex and lengthy, requiring specialist assessment skills. The techniques of photoplethysmography and air plethysmography are excellent non-invasive tests but are limited to the field of research due to complexity and time required to complete the assessement[13,14]. Ambulatory venous pressure analysis is the gold standard for assessing the venous flow in a leg, however it is an invasive test, complex and time-consuming[13]. These assessments provide value for researchers investigating haemodynamic responses to treatment, and for advancing techniques in the long-term[15].

Clinical

Clinical assessment in varicose vein treatment is crucial to delineating disease and assessing disease progression and resolution, but does not attempt to truly investigate symptomatology[16-18]. The Clinical Etiological Anatomical Pathological (CEAP) scoring system is a static system, designed to categorise patients into distinct clinical stages[18]. Movement between stages is slow and it has been formulated as an "entry point" score, and so is not suitable for dynamic assessment post-treatment, though it is often quoted. C0 represents no venous disease, through to C6 representing an active venous ulcer. Advanced CEAP scoring allows all parts of the clinical situation to be described, in theory allowing complete reconstruction of the disease. However this is complex both in construction and interpretation and so often only the maximum Clinical (C) stage is described and quoted. The Venous Clinical Severity Score (VCSS)[17] is a more dynamic score, and allows for better symptomatic and functional description of the problem. However, without careful symptom assessment this does not tell the whole story. These scores can be described as Clinical Reported Outcome Measures - CROMs.

Functional

The symptoms of varicose veins affects a patient's life, however so do many other conditions and confounding factors. Therefore an appropriate starting point for assessment would be to measure the patient's quality of life. These assessments utilise Patient Reported Outcome Measures - PROMs. It is now recognised that in order to drive forward the quality of patient-centred care, these measures are crucial[19].

Generic

Work based in Occupational Health Medicine have tried to quantify health status for the past 30 years[20,21]. This has led to patient completed generic health questionnaires such as the Nottingham Health Profile or the General Health Questionnaire, which provided patient reported measures of their health at that point. Further development led to quality of life tools such as the Short Form 36 (SF36) questionnaire series[22] or the EuroQol 5 Domain questionnaire (EQ-5D). These assess the World Health Organisation's definition of health - "Health is a state of complete physical, mental and social well-being and not merely the absence of disease or infirmity". These global scores of health allow clinicians to assess treatments and stages of clinical disease - such as how does a patient with Clinical Venous Disease stage 3 feel overall[18]?

Crucially, generic quality of life measures allow the calculation of health economics measures such as Cost Effectiveness, Cost Benefit, Cost Minimization and Cost Utility. This allows the calculation of benefit to the population as a whole, and is crucial in nationalised health care services such as the National Health Service in the United Kingdom.

Specific

Generic health questionnaires offer validated objective methods of scoring a persons symptoms related to the disease in question. Multiple options exist for this as well, with the most popular English language questionnaire being the Aberdeen Varicose Vein Questionnaire (AVVQ)[23] and the most popular French language one being the ChronIc Venous Insufficiency Questionnaire (CIVIQ)[24]. These are once again patient reported questionnaires, or PROMs[25], and provide key indicators of the symptomatic benefit obtained by treating patients. The AVVQ is a 13 question combined drawing and question survey, with the CIVIQ being 20 questions with tick boxes only. These surveys delineate and respond appropriately to venous disease and have recently shown to be very well correlated to each other by our group[26]. This reinforces their suitability for symptom measurement, and they are also correlated with the generic quality of life outcomes. Previous work in our unit has also compared the Specific Quality of Life and Outcome Response-Venous (SQOR-V)[27]. An alternative option is the Venous Insufficiency Epidemiological and Economic Study Quality of Life/Symptoms questionnaire (VEINES-QOL/Sym) though the 26 item questionnaire is less well represented in the published literature[28].

Our unit has shown correlations between the specific and generic QOL tools, though this is only of moderate strength[26,27]. Both of these outcomes are expected.

Recent work has led to the development of the VVSymQ, a questionnaire which utilises a digital delivery system to allow immediate reporting and calculation. The studies describing its development highlight reasonable correlations with the other main specific quality of life assessments[29].

To review the outcomes of a treatment designed to improve symptoms, PROMs are vital, as they provide a method of quantifying and standardising outcomes between patients, centres and treatments beyond that provided by levels of satisfaction[30,31].

Hospital Episode Statistics (HES) Data and National Patient Reported Outcomes

In the United Kingdom (UK), all National Health Service (NHS) patients undergoing varicose vein treatment since 2009 are encouraged to fill in NHS PROMs which include the EQ-5D and the AVVQ, and in addition to more general questions on satisfaction and post-operative complications. These are completed pre-operatively and 3-6 months post-operatively. This has allowed the generation of a large databank showing the outcomes of venous surgery from a national perspective[32].

Currently available data (2015-2016) shows good improvements throughout the UK with an average improvement of 38% in AVVQ scores with 83% of patients improving and 10% in EQ-5D Index with 53% of patients improving[32,33].

Previous work by Nesbitt et al. analysed the HES PROM data from 2009-2010 and found similar figures, with an average improvement of 43% in AVVQ, but only 5% in EQ-5D. 85% of patients deemed their outcome as good or better, and 90% had an improvement in symptoms. Work by Moore et al. assessing the burden of primary varicose vein disease in Europe[34] found that, in the national statistics available at least, there was a marked disparity between patients treated and the level at which treatment appears to be offered.

Modelling of outcomes

The use of these tools allow us to perform advanced modelling methods on the patient data. Carradice et al. have completed extensive modelling work on the patient and clinician reported outcome measures above[35]. This allowed the unveiling of significant quality of life impairments in patients with C2-4 disease, without any significant difference between groups, though as the stages increased in severity so did the QOL deficit. This work identified that patients with varicose veins have similar bodily pain scores as recent myocardial infarction patients, and chronic physical dysfunction in line with congestive cardiac failure patients.

Guidelines

With all of these measures available, how does one assess which to report? Guidelines issued in 2007 and 2009 by the American Venous Forum have been adopted in many countries[36]. These guidelines are aimed at the endovenous revolution, dealing specifically with thermal ablation techniques; however, the perioperative and follow-up care advice is appropriate and key and transferable to both non-thermal ablation techniques and open surgery.

Heterogeneity

Despite the guidelines of the American Venous Forum being available for 6 years[36] many studies are still not reporting as one would hope[37]. This leads to difficulty in assessing the research body as a whole. However, as the guidelines disseminate it is hoped that newer studies will report completely, and indeed recent publications are doing so - for example Rasmussen et al.'s study investigating 4 separate treatment modalities[38]. The publication of comparable randomised studies in addition to the growing NHS HES PROMs data set allows confidence in the generalisability of such results[39].

Conclusion

Assessing the success of varicose vein surgery is a complex and important part of the phlebologist's practice. It must be done robustly in order to provide the clinician with confidence that their treatment is beneficial and also to allow experience of the variable nature of outcomes from venous disease. Whilst technical details and assessment is a useful component to assess treatment, PROMs are the only method of obtaining symptomatic outcomes - crucial in the treatment of a symptomatic but benign disease that is extremely common, but subject to great and complex variation.

References

1. Neglén P, Egger JF III, Olivier J, Raju S. Hemodynamic and clinical impact of ultrasound-derived venous reflux parameters. JVS. Elsevier; 2004;40(2):303–10.
2. Bradbury A, Evans C, Allan P, Lee A, Ruckley CV, Fowkes FG. What are the symptoms of varicose veins? Edinburgh vein study cross sectional population survey. BMJ. 1999 Feb 6;318(7180):353–6.
3. Allan PL, Bradbury AW, Evans CJ, Lee AJ, Vaughan Ruckley C, Fowkes FG. Patterns of reflux and severity of varicose veins in the general population--Edinburgh Vein Study. EJVES. 2000 Nov;20(5):470–7.
4. Lane TRA, Shepherd AC, Gohel MS, Franklin IJ, Davies AH. Big Veins, Big Deal - Vein Diameter Affects Disease Severity, not Quality of Life. JVS:VLD. Elsevier Inc; 2013 Jan 1;1(1):101.

5.	NHS North West London. Planned Procedures with a Threshold - Varicose Veins [Internet]. 0 ed. London, UK: NHS North West London; 2011. Available from: http://www.westminster. nhs.uk/English/about-us/northwestlondon/Pages/ifrservice.aspx

6.	Van Den Bos RR, Arends L, Kockaert M, Neumann M, Nijsten T. Endovenous therapies of lower extremity varicosities: a meta-analysis. JVS. 2009 Jan 1;49(1):230–9.

7.	Siribumrungwong B, Noorit P, Wilasrusmee C, Attia J, Thakkinstian A. A Systematic Review and Meta-analysis of Randomised Controlled Trials Comparing Endovenous Ablation and Surgical Intervention in Patients with Varicose Vein. 2012 Jun 13;44(2):214–23.

8.	Shepherd AC, Gohel MS, Lim CS, Hamish M, Davies AH. The treatment of varicose veins: an investigation of patient preferences and expectations. Phlebology. 2010 Apr;25(2):54–65.

9.	Pichot O, Kabnick LS, Creton D, Merchant RF, Schuller-Petroviae S, Chandler JG. Duplex ultrasound scan findings two years after great saphenous vein radiofrequency endovenous obliteration. J Vasc Surg. 2004 Jan;39(1):189–95.

10.	Salles-Cunha SX, Comerota AJ, Tzilinis A, Dosick SM, Gale SS, Seiwert AJ, et al. Ultrasound findings after radiofrequency ablation of the great saphenous vein: Descriptive analysis. J Vasc Surg. 2004 Dec;40(6):1166–73.

11.	Lurie F, Creton D, Eklöf B, Kabnick LS, Kistner RL, Pichot O, et al. Prospective randomised study of endovenous radiofrequency obliteration (closure) versus ligation and vein stripping (EVOLVeS): two-year follow-up. EJVES. 2005 Jan;29(1):67–73.

12.	Gohel MS, Davies AH. Choosing between varicose vein treatments: looking beyond occlusion rates. Phlebology. 2008 Apr 1;23(2):51–2.

13.	Marston WA. PPG, APG, duplex: Which noninvasive tests are most appropriate for the management of patients with chronic venous insufficiency? Elsevier; 2002 Mar;15(1):13–20.

14.	Lurie F, Rooke TW. Evaluation of venous function by indirect non-invasive testing (plethysmography). In: Gloviczki P, editor. Handbook of venous disorders: Guidelines of the American Venous Forum. 3rd ed. London: Hodder Arnold; 2007. pp. 156–9.

15.	Lattimer CR, Azzam M, Kalodiki E, Geroulakos G. Quantifying saphenous recirculation in patients with primary lower extremity venous reflux. J Vasc Surg :VLD. 2015.

16.	Gloviczki P, Gloviczki ML. Guidelines for the management of varicose veins. Phlebology. 2012 Feb 6;27(Supplement 1):2–9.

17.	Vasquez MA, Rabe E, McLafferty RB, Shortell CK, Marston WA, Gillespie D, et al. Revision of the venous clinical severity score: venous outcomes consensus statement: special communication of the American Venous Forum Ad Hoc Outcomes Working Group. J Vasc Surg. 2010 Nov;52(5):1387–96.

18.	Eklöf BG, Rutherford RB, Bergan JJ, Carpentier PH, Gloviczki P, Kistner RL, et al. Revision of the CEAP classification for chronic venous disorders: consensus statement. JVS [Internet]. 2004 Dec;40(6):1248–52. Available from: http://www.sciencedirect.com/science/article/pii/ S0741521404012777

19.	Black N. Patient reported outcome measures could help transform healthcare. 2013 Jan

28;346(jan28 1):f167–7.

20. Hunt SM, McEwen J. The development of a subjective health indicator. 1980 Nov;2(3):231–46.

21. McKenna SP, Payne RL. Comparison of the General Health Questionnaire and the Nottingham Health Profile in a Study of Unemployed and Re-Employed Men. 1989;6(1):3–8.

22. Ware JE Jr, Sherbourne CD. The MOS 36-item short-form health survey (SF-36): I. Conceptual framework and item selection. 1992 Jun;30(6):473–83.

23. Garratt AM, Macdonald LM, Ruta DA, Russell IT, Buckingham JK, Krukowski ZH. Towards measurement of outcome for patients with varicose veins. Qual Health Care. 1993 Mar;2(1):5–10.

24. Launois R, Reboul-Marty J, Henry B. Construction and validation of a quality of life questionnaire in chronic lower limb venous insufficiency (CIVIQ). Qual Life Res. 1996 Dec;5(6):539–54.

25. Ousey K, Cook L. Understanding patient reported outcome measures (PROMs). Br J Community Nurs. 2011 Feb;16(2):80–2.

26. Kuet ML, Lane TRA, Franklin IJ, Davies AH. A Study To Compare Disease Specific Quality Of Life Scoring Systems In Patients With Varicose Veins. Phoenix, USA; 2013.

27. Shepherd AC, Gohel MS, Lim CS, Davies AH. A study to compare disease-specific quality of life with clinical anatomical and hemodynamic assessments in patients with varicose veins. J Vasc Surg. 2011 Feb;53(2):374–82.

28. Lamping DL, Schroter S, Kurz X, Kahn SR, Abenhaim LA. Evaluation of outcomes in chronic venous disorders of the leg: development of a scientifically rigorous, patient-reported measure of symptoms and quality of life. J Vasc Surg. 2003 Feb;37(2):410–9.

29. Wright DDI, Paty J, Turner-Bowker DM. Psychometric Evaluation of a New Patient-Reported Outcome (PRO) Symptom Diary for Varicose Veins: VVSymQ(®) Instrument. Patient. 2016 Mar 25.

30. Davies AH, Steffen C, Cosgrove C, Wilkins DC. Varicose vein surgery: patient satisfaction. J R Coll Surg Edinb. 1995 Oct;40(5):298–9.

31. Campbell WB, Vijay Kumar A, Collin TW, Allington KL, Michaels JA. The outcome of varicose vein surgery at 10 years: clinical findings, symptoms and patient satisfaction. Ann R Coll Surg Engl. 2003 Jan 1;85(1):52–7.

32. NHS Digital. Provisional Monthly Patient Reported Outcome Measures (PROMs) in England. The Health and Social Care Information Centre, NHS; 2017.

33. Hospital Episode Statistics Online [Internet]. NHS Digital, NHS; 2017 [cited 2017 May 30]. Available from: http://content.digital.nhs.uk/searchcatalogue

34. Moore HM, Lane TRA, Thapar A, Franklin IJ, Davies AH. The European burden of primary varicose veins. Phlebology. 2013 Mar;28(Suppl 1):141–7.

35. Carradice D, Mazari FAK, Samuel N, Allgar V, Hatfield J, Chetter IC. Modelling the effect

of venous disease on quality of life. Br J Surg. 2011 Aug;98(8):1089–98.

36.   Kundu S, Lurie F, Millward SF, Padberg F, Vedantham S, Elias SM, et al. Recommended reporting standards for endovenous ablation for the treatment of venous insufficiency: joint statement of the American Venous Forum and the Society of Interventional Radiology. J Vasc Surg. 2007; 46 (3):582-9.

37.   Thakur B, Shalhoub J, Hill AM, Gohel MS, Davies AH. Heterogeneity of reporting standards in randomised clinical trials of endovenous interventions for varicose veins. Eur J Vasc Endovasc Surg. 2010 Oct;40(4):528–33.

38.   Rasmussen LH, Lawaetz M, Bjoern L, Vennits B, Blemings A, Eklöf B. Randomized clinical trial comparing endovenous laser ablation, radiofrequency ablation, foam sclerotherapy and surgical stripping for great saphenous varicose veins. Br J Surg. 2011 Aug;98(8):1079–87.

39.   Black N. Why we need observational studies to evaluate the effectiveness of health care. BMJ Group; 1996 May 11;312(7040):1215.

Chapter 15

Transvaginal Duplex Ultrasound Scanning for Diagnosis of Pelvic Vein Reflux

Author
Judith M Holdstock

Institution
The Whiteley Clinic, Stirling House, Stirling Road, Guildford, Surrey GU2 7RF

Introduction

Over the last fifteen years the treatment options for varicose veins have undergone radical and progressive change. There has been a corresponding evolution in the diagnosis of venous reflux patterns to maximise the advantages of the new, minimally invasive, treatments available. Duplex ultrasound for leg varicose veins has commonly been restricted to examination of the major trunks, the Great and Small Saphenous veins. However to aid successful customised treatment of varicose veins a more detailed duplex ultrasound scan is required looking at tributaries, perforator veins and complex patterns of veins. This has been termed an 'extended reflux scan'. Early in our Clinics' fifteen year history of varicose vein treatment, we noted some patients presenting with complex patterns of varicose veins on the inner or posterior aspect of the upper thigh communicating internally into the labial region and pelvis. Our experience showed that despite successful laser or radiofrequency ablation of truncal veins and perforators with avulsion of varices, there was a tendency to prompt recurrence of varicose veins in these patients from the pelvic element. It was a natural progression to perform a transvaginal duplex ultrasound scan to look for the source of reflux in the pelvis and identify which veins were causing these atypical leg varicose veins. Initially our intention to treat the pelvic veins was purely to facilitate better treatment of the leg varicose veins. However, we found that a percentage of our patients also reported resolution of a range of symptoms associated with 'Pelvic congestion syndrome'. Our experience with diagnosis and treatment of pelvic vein reflux over the last fifteen years has built an extensive library of the common patterns of pelvic reflux, their associated varices and symptoms and the prevalence with which this occurs.

Leg Vein patterns associated with pelvic vein reflux

While some varicose veins, arising from the pelvis, may be clinically apparent, the majority are discovered during duplex ultrasound examination of their leg vein reflux pattern. The pelvic vein component may be the predominant cause of leg vein reflux in some cases. However, it is frequently seen as an adjunctive component of a wider pattern of venous incompetence. It is frequently overlooked in the presence of concurrent truncal saphenous reflux patterns, which likely accounts for its higher incidence in those presenting with recurrent varicose veins.

The following examples show some of the more clinically obvious varicose vein patterns associated with pelvic vein reflux.

Varicose veins on the proximal inner thigh lying posterior to the adductor longus tendon (Figure 1)

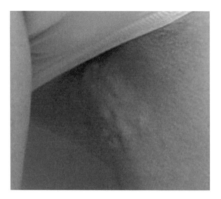

Figure 1: Clinical picture of female patient with varicose veins on proximal inner thigh – para-vulval varicose veins. Typical of patients with leg varicose veins with a significant pelvic component.

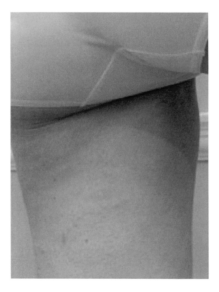

Figure 2: Clinical picture of a female patient with varicose veins on proximal posterior/ lateral thigh arising from para-vulval or perineal regions. This diagonal pattern of varicose veins winding around the thigh from upper inner to lower outer is typical of patients with leg varicose veins with a significant pelvic component.

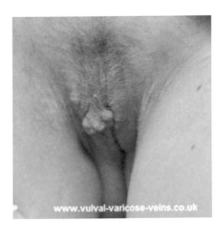

Figure 3: Clinical picture showing vulval varices (Grade 4 - see Table 1)

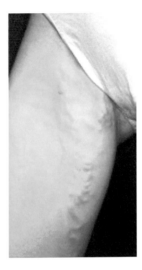

Figure 4: Clinical picture of a female patient with large recurrent varicose veins clinically arising from two different areas – the groin from neovascular tissue following a previous high saphenous tie, and also from the para-vulvar veins suggesting a significant component of the venous reflux is from pelvic venous reflux.

Varicose veins, arising from the posterior vulva and perianal region, travelling across the posterior thigh or buttock crease and lateral aspect of the thigh, often associated with thread vein formation on the lateral aspect of the thigh (Figure 2).

Varicose veins lying within, the vaginal wall or vulva and labium. These may be symptomatic and clinically obvious as in (Figure 3). Some may have been noticeable during pregnancy but less so post-partum, although many remain symptomatic especially during menstruation. Recurrent varicose vein patterns from pelvic vein origin may be seen after previous sapheno-femoral junction (SFJ) ligation and/or stripping. These may be seen communicating with remnants of un-stripped Great Saphenous vein (GSV) or revascularisation of strip tracks in previously stripped GSV. They may also be associated with neo-vascular tissue at the groin resulting from previous SFJ ligation (Figure 4).

153

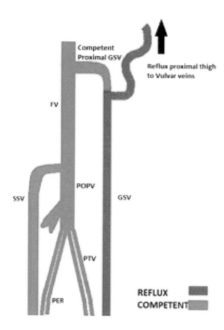

Figure 5: Diagram showing a possible pattern of pelvic vein reflux associated with leg varicose veins. The descending incompetent tributary (usually seen clinically as a para-vulval varicose vein) bypasses the competent SFJ and proximal competent GSV, refluxing into an incompetent GSV trunk.

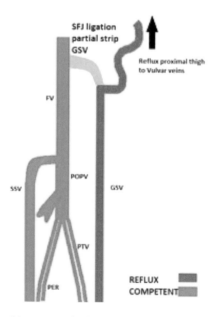

Figure 6: Diagram showing a possible pattern of pelvic vein reflux associated with recurrent leg varicose veins. A descending incompetent tributary (usually seen clinically as a para-vulval varicose vein) connects onto the incompetent GSV, after SFJ ligation. This is a common pattern of recurrent varicose veins as, in the past, few doctors have recognised the contribution of pelvic venous reflux in such patients.

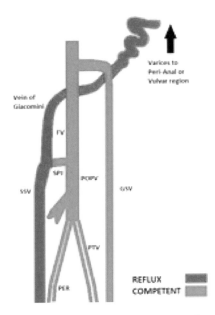

Figure 7: Diagram showing a possible pattern of pelvic vein reflux associated with leg varicose veins. Incompetent peri-anal varices can connect onto the Giacomini vein and be associated with SSV reflux.

Other patterns of leg vein reflux with an associated pelvic component may not be obvious on clinical examination. However, anyone familiar with venous incompetence scanning of the legs may encounter certain 'atypical' patterns of reflux which may indicate pelvic vein involvement.

Figure 5 represents a pattern of reflux, where the SFJ and proximal 5-10cm of the GSV are competent. There is a tortuous vein extending from the vulvar area down to the GSV which demonstrates reflux distal to this confluence. This is a relatively common pattern and is often a source of recurrent varicose veins where the SFJ has been ligated without complete stripping of the GSV Figure 6.

Varicose veins in the peri-anal region can communicate directly with the vein of Giacomini on the posterior aspect of the thigh and be associated with corresponding reflux in the SSV as seen in Figure 7.

There are numerous variations of leg vein reflux patterns which can have a major or minor contribution from the pelvic veins. At our clinic, it has become standard practice to look for any communications to the pelvic veins as an integral part of all extended venous reflux ultrasound scans.

Prevalence of pelvic vein reflux and reflux patterns

Our unit has previously shown that between 15-20% of women presenting with leg varicose veins[1] have an underlying pattern associated with pelvic vein incompetence with the figure being somewhat higher in female patients with recurrent varicose veins where the incidence is up to 30%[2].

A recent audit was carried out over a single year series (2011). All new female patients attending the clinic for the first time were included in the series, a total of 593 patients. Of these 153 patients

(25.8%) were found to have a leg vein pattern with communication to the pelvis and all of these proceeded to have a transvaginal duplex scan. Figure 8 and 9 demonstrate both the incidence of reflux found in the four pelvic trunks and also the most common patterns of reflux identified in the pelvis.

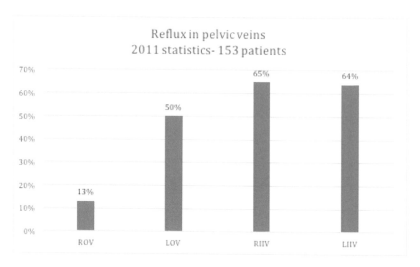

Figure 8: Graph showing the reflux in each of the pelvic veins that was identified in 153/593 (25.8%) patients in a clinical audit conducted in 2011.

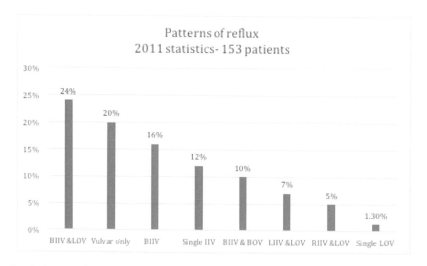

Figure 9: Graph showing the incidence of pelvic vein reflux patterns that were identified in all patients with incompetent pelvic veins identified in the 2011 audit.

Note that isolated left ovarian vein reflux is present in only 1.3% of the females in this group.

Also of interest is that 20% of patients show reflux only in their vulvar region without significant pelvic truncal involvement. This sub-group was largely composed of either nulliparous women, those with single parity status or ladies who had undergone hysterectomy. In the nulliparous and single parity group it is possible this pattern is indicative of ascending reflux from the legs into the vulvar veins.

Symptoms associated with pelvic vein reflux

'Pelvic congestion syndrome' (PCS) is a term used to label a variety of symptoms associated with reflux in the pelvic veins. The presence of often large varices in the pelvis can cause pressure and inflammation in the pelvis and have an effect on the bladder and bowel in addition to the uterus and ovaries.

Symptoms such as throbbing and aching in the pelvis or lower back, especially after prolonged periods of standing can be experienced. These symptoms can increase in the pre-menstrual and menstruating phase of the female cycle. Irritable bowel syndrome, bladder frequency and irritation, pain on intercourse (dyspareunia) are often experienced. It is not uncommon to find polycystic ovaries (PCO) in patients who experience pelvic vein reflux.

Not all patients who have leg varicose vein patterns associated with pelvic vein reflux exhibit all or any of the symptoms of pelvic congestion although they do often experience 'restless legs', aching and throbbing in their leg varicose veins and thread veins, these symptoms are exacerbated with cyclical changes, especially menstruation. Indeed these patterns are often much more symptomatic than varicose veins arising from saphenous vein origin.

Which Pelvic veins can be involved in Pelvic reflux patterns and how does this relate to the symptoms experienced?

Pelvic vein reflux has been mainly thought to be due to the left ovarian vein 'nutcracker' effect due to compression of the left renal and ovarian vein. Up until now methods of imaging the pelvic veins, either contrast venography, CT or MRI imaging rely heavily on 'size' and dilation of veins rather than functional reflux imaging and have given limited information regarding patterns of pelvic vein incompetence. This has resulted largely in treatment of only the ovarian veins (predominantly the left).

However, transvaginal duplex ultrasound can give both anatomical and functional information. In close detail, the relationships between the four main pelvic trunks and associated varices can be examined and all relevant trunks, tributaries and varices tested for reflux, dilation and syphon effects. Varices can be seen in the ovarian vein plexus but can also be noted in the uterine plexus, with dilation of the arcuate veins in the uterine wall. Varices are also common in the vaginal wall, in the peri-urethral area, peri-anal area and vulvar veins. Most importantly these varices appear to be associated not only with the ovarian veins but also with reflux in tributaries of the internal iliac veins such as those draining the bladder, urethral area, bowel, rectum and uterine area plus veins communicating with the thigh and buttocks such as the obturator, pudendal and inferior gluteal veins (from the anterior trunk of the internal iliac vein) and the ilio-lumbar, sacral and superior gluteal (from the posterior trunk of the internal iliac vein). Distribution of varices, around the urethra and base of the bladder, are often linked to symptoms of irritable bladder, urinary frequency and urge incontinence. Internal iliac vein tributaries may be seen communicating with peri-anal varices and often directly into haemorrhoids.

What can be seen on transvaginal duplex ultrasound imaging?

Grayscale 'B mode' imaging allows interrogation of the pelvic anatomy and identification of the ovarian veins and internal iliac veins, tributaries and associated varicose veins. Evaluation of reflux within the pelvic venous trunks and varices can be performed using colour flow and spectral Doppler with the subject placed in a semi-erect position with their head and torso elevated to 45 degrees and

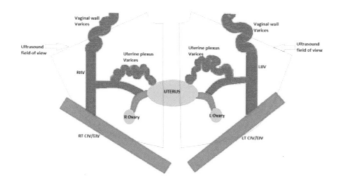

Figure 10: Diagram of what can be observed with a transvaginal ultrasound scan when examining the internal iliac veins and associated veins.

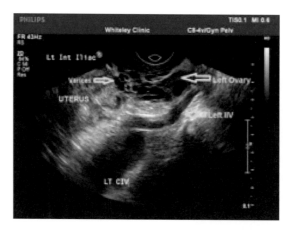

Figure 11: Transvaginal ultrasound scan (greyscale) showing left common and internal iliac veins as well as associated varices.

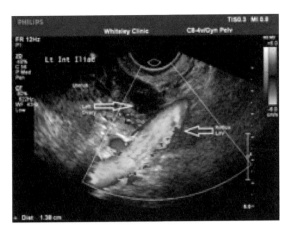

Figure 12: Transvaginal duplex ultrasound scan with colour flow Doppler showing gross reflux in the left internal iliac vein.

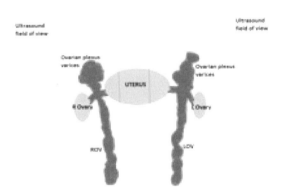

Figure 13: Diagram of the anatomy of the ovarian veins as related to transvaginal duplex ultrasound.

employing a Valsalva breathing technique to place pressure on the venous system and identify flow reversal and venous distension.

Coronal (transverse) and coronal/oblique images achieve the best views of the internal iliac and ovarian veins.

Obtaining views of the Internal Iliac veins:

With the transducer angled into the lateral fornix in coronal/oblique plane the Internal Iliac veins which lie on the side wall of the pelvis, lateral to the uterus and ovaries can be identified (Figure 10).

The left internal iliac vein can be identified arising from the common/external iliac veins and traveling along the pelvic side wall lateral to the ovary and traveling directly towards the transducer as shown in the grayscale image (Figure 11) with reflux demonstrated within the left internal iliac vein colour flow Doppler in (Figure 12).

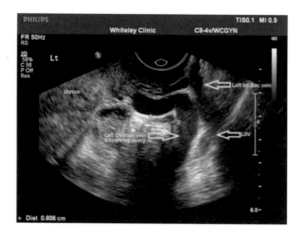

Figure 14: Transvaginal ultrasound scan (greyscale) showing left ovarian and internal iliac veins.

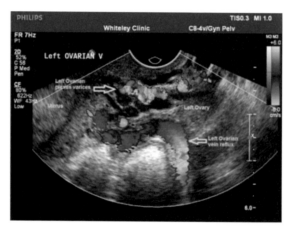

Figure 15: Transvaginal duplex ultrasound showing reflux in the left ovarian vein and the left ovarian venous plexus.

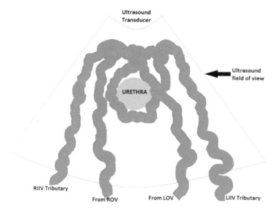

Figure 16: Diagram of peri-urethral varicose veins as related to transvaginal duplex ultrasound.

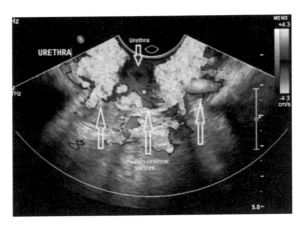

Figure 17: Transvaginal scan showing peri-urethral varicose veins that can be compared directly with the diagram Figure 16.

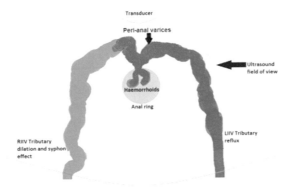

Figure 18: A diagram of the communication between peri-anal varicose veins and haemorrhoids as related to transvaginal duplex ultrasound.

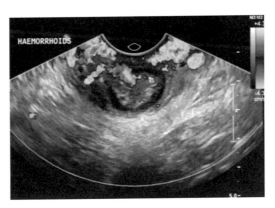

Figure 19: Transvaginal scan showing communication between peri-anal varicose veins and haemorrhoids that can be compared directly with the diagram Figure 19.

	Description	Frequency seen at present
Grade 0	Normal – no varicosities nor venous reflux in vulva	Usual
Grade 1	No visible varicosities in vulva, but ultrasound proven reflux in vulval veins usually with para-vulval varicose veins seen on inner thigh	Common – 1 in 5 females presenting with primary varicose veins of the legs
Grade 2	Visible varicosities seen through mucosa of inner labia and lover vagina and ultrasound proven reflux in vulval veins.	Uncommon
Grade 3	Isolated varicosities seen on standing through skin of outer labia majora without a distortion of the general anatomy of the area	Very uncommon
Grade 4	Extensive varicosities of the labia, distorting skin and distorting the gross anatomy of the area on standing	Rare

Table 1: Table of The Whiteley Clinic grading system used for Varicose Veins of the Vulva. The assessment is made in a non-pregnant state and when standing. Frequency may be underestimated as this has been assessed on those finding that something can be done, despite the usual advice to the contrary. First published: MS Whiteley. The treatment of varicose veins of the vulva and vagina. In: Greenhalgh RM (Ed.) Vascular and Endovascular Controversies Update. London Biba Publishing, 2012 p. 666-670

Obtaining views of the ovarian veins:

The Ovarian veins lie medial to the Internal Iliac veins and typically lie sandwiched between the uterus and ovaries (Figure 13). The left ovarian vein can be seen in Figure 14 traversing the left ovary. Note the relationship to the left Internal Iliac vein lying lateral to the ovarian vein on the left sidewall of the pelvis. Reflux within the left ovarian vein and associate ovarian plexus varices can be seen in Figure 15.

Anterior vaginal wall, peri-urethral varicose veins and pudendal communicating veins can be identified on a coronal view with the transducer positioned just inside the vagina and angled anteriorly towards the symphysis pubis (Figure 16 and 17).

When the transducer is angled, from this position, posteriorly towards the rectum, communicating tributaries from the internal iliac veins, peri-anal varicose veins and haemorrhoids can be identified (Figure 18 and 19).

The Whiteley Clinic protocol for assessing pelvic vein incompetence

Over the last fifteen years we have developed and refined the Holdstock/Harrison protocol, in use at The Whiteley Clinic, for the assessment of pelvic vein reflux and for gauging the severity and extent of the reflux pattern.

The key points we look for are:

a) Reflux of greater than 1 second within venous trunks, effectively the reflux should last until the end of the Valsalva.

b) The trunk diameter will generally be greater than 5mm. However, smaller trunks with persistent reflux can be considered.

c) The venous trunks should exhibit dilation on Valsalva in addition to reflux.

d) There may be contra-lateral dilation and syphon effects between right and left ovarian veins and right and left internal iliac veins or ipsi-lateral syphon between the ovarian and internal iliac trunks. Syphon effects are noted when reflux is so great in one vein that it sets up a corresponding suction effect with massively increased antegrade flow in the opposing trunk when Valsalva is performed.

e) Associated varices should exhibit distension and flow reversal on Valsalva.

Reflux can be graded on a scale of one to four, where:

1) Minor or trickle reflux
2) Moderate reflux
3) Severe or marked reflux
4) Gross reflux

The severity of the pelvic vein incompetence also depends on the number of pelvic trunks involved and also the size of the pelvic trunks and associated varices.

When gauging severity we also take into account any symptoms, either in the legs or pelvis experienced by the patient. We take a detailed obstetric and gynaecological history.

This should include:

Number of pregnancies and mode of delivery, normal vaginal delivery or trial of labour and elective caesarean section. We also note any history of gynaecological surgery.

We document symptoms such as back pain, worsening over the course of the day, irritable bladder or urinary frequency/urge incontinence, irritable bowel symptoms, haemorrhoids, dyspareunia, cyclical symptoms or dragging sensation in the vulvar/labial area, leg symptoms worsening during menstruation and note any obvious visible varicose veins on the vaginal wall or labia.

Does this problem only occur in women?

Whilst the majority of our experience is concerned with diagnosis of pelvic vein reflux in women we do encounter some men who possess complex leg varicose vein patterns arising from the pelvis. It is relatively simple to confirm or exclude reflux in the testicular veins by performing duplex ultrasound of these veins within the scrotal sac, inguinal canal and abdomen. Unfortunately, we have found trans-abdominal pelvic ultrasound of limited use in diagnosing reflux within the internal iliac veins. We are currently exploring other options for imaging the male pelvis and hope to be able to share our experience in the near future.

Conclusion

I hope this chapter has shed some light on this largely overlooked causal element of venous reflux, both in relation to the diagnosis and management of leg varicose veins and also to the symptoms women experience with pelvic congestion syndrome.

References

1. Marsh P, Holdstock J, Harrison C, Smith C, Price BA, Whiteley MS. Pelvic vein reflux in female patients with varicose veins: comparison of incidence between a specialist private vein clinic and the vascular department of a National Health Service District General Hospital. Phlebology. 2009; 24 (3): 108-13.

2. Whiteley AM, Taylor DC, Whiteley MS. Pelvic Venous Reflux is a Major Contributory Cause of Recurrent Varicose Veins in more than a Quarter of Women. J Vasc Surg Venous Lymphat Disord. 2013; 1 (1): 100-101.

3. Kurklinsky AK, Rooke TW. Nutcracker Phenomenon and Nutcracker Syndrome. Mayo Clin Proc. 2010; 85 (6): 552-9.

4. Rudloff U, Holmes RJ, Prem JT, Faust GR, Moldwin R, Siegel D. Mesoaortic compression of the left renal vein (nutcracker syndrome): case reports and review of the literature. Ann Vasc Surg. 2006; 20 (1): 120-9.

5. S Takebayashi, T Ueki, N Ikeda and A Fujikawa. Diagnosis of the nutcracker syndrome with color Doppler sonography: correlation with flow patterns on retrograde left renal venography. AJR Am J Roentgenology. 1999; 172 (1): 39-42

6. Rogers A, Beech A, Braithwaite B. Transperitoneal laparoscopic left gonadal vein ligation can be the right treatment option for pelvic congestion symptoms secondary to nutcracker syndrome. Vascular. 2007; 15 (4): 238-40.

7. Ignacio EA, Dua R, Sarin S, Harper AS, Yim D, Mathur V, Venbrux AC. Pelvic Congestion Syndrome: Diagnosis and Treatment. Seminars in Interventional Radiology. 2008; 25 (4): 361-368.

8. Hocquelet A, Le Bras Y, Balian E, Bouzgarrou M, Meyer M, Rigou G, Grenier N. Evaluation of the efficacy of endovascular treatment of pelvic congestion syndrome. Diagn Interv Imaging. 2014; 95 (3): 301-6.

9. Laborda A, Medrano J, de Blas I, Urtiaga I, Carnevale FC, de Gregorio MA. Endovascular treatment of pelvic congestion syndrome: visual analog scale (VAS) long-term follow-up clinical evaluation in 202 patients. Cardiovasc Intervent Radiol. 201;36(4):1006-14. doi:

10.1007/s00270-013-0586-2. Epub 2013 Mar 2.

10. Cho SJ, Lee TH, Shim KY, Hong SS, Goo DE. Pelvic congestion syndrome diagnosed using endoscopic ultrasonography. Phlebology. 2014; 29(2): 126-8.

11. Meneses L, Fava M, Diaz P, Andía M, Tejos C, Irarrazaval P, Uribe S. Embolization of incompetent pelvic veins for the treatment of recurrent varicose veins in lower limbs and pelvic congestion syndrome. Cardiovasc Intervent Radiol. 2013;36(2):565.

12. Kies DD, Kim HS. Pelvic congestion syndrome: a review of current diagnostic and minimally invasive treatment modalities. Phlebology. 2012; 27 (1): 52-7

13. Jin KN, Lee W, Jae HJ, Yin YH, Chung JW, Park JH. Venous reflux from the pelvis and vulvoperineal region as a possible cause of lower extremity varicose veins: diagnosis with computed tomographic and ultrasonographic findings. J Comput Assist Tomogr. 2009; 33(5): 763-9.

Chapter 16

Treatment of Symptomatic Venous Reflux in the Ovarian and Internal Iliac Veins by Catheter Embolisation

Author
Previn Diwakar

Institution
The Whiteley Clinic, Stirling House, Stirling Road, Guildford, Surrey GU2 7RF

Introduction

Pelvic venous incompetence (PVI) is defined as venous reflux in the ovarian, internal iliac or parauterine veins. The reflux may or may not result in increased venous engorgement (i.e. congestion) and subsequently the term PVI is now considered more appropriate than the older term pelvic congestion syndrome (PCS). It can present as either atypical primary or recurrent leg varices, or chronic pelvic pain.

The incidence of recurrence following surgical management of varicose veins ranges from 20-80%[1-5]. There is a high incidence of PVI in patients presenting with atypical recurrent varicose veins arising on the buttocks, upper posteromedial thigh and extending to the vulval and perivulval regions[6]. Chronic pelvic pain (CPP) is defined as noncyclic pain originating in the lower abdomen or pelvis for more than 6 months[7] and up to 39.1% of women can be affected by it at some time in their lives[8].

Pathophysiology

Although first described as far back as 1857[9], it wasn't until the 1920's that ovarian varicosities were associated with CPP[10]. There are numerous theories as to the precise aetiology of pelvic varicosities. Damaged or absent valves are significant in the development of retrograde flow[10] and the capacity of the ovarian veins can increase greatly in pregnancy with pelvic varicosities significantly more likely in multiparous women[11]. The ovarian veins are exposed to a 100-fold increased concentration of oestrogens compared to the peripheral venous circulation leading to the theory that hormonal factors play a part in the development of the varicosities of the ovarian vein. This is supported by the fact that PVI primarily affects pre-menopausal women. Other anatomical causes for the development of PVI, reported in the literature include uterine malposition, renal "nutcracker" syndrome, portal hypertension, iliac compression syndrome (May-Thurner syndrome) and inferior vena cava syndrome[12-16].

Clinical presentation
PVI typically, though not exclusively, presents in pre-menopausal multiparous women. They may present with recurrent leg varicosities and/or atypical varicose veins arising on the buttock or upper posteromedial thigh and extending to the vulval and peri-vulval region with or without concurrent chronic pelvic pain. The pelvic pain is usually described as a deep, dull pelvic ache, dyspareunia or post-coital pain centred around the lower pelvis, vulva and upper thighs, exacerbated by prolonged standing or an increase in intra-abdominal pressure (straining or lifting). The pain is typically worse at the end of the day, immediately pre-menstrual or during pregnancy. Some patients describe the pain worsening with each subsequent pregnancy.

Anatomy
Pelvic venous drainage is via 3 main pairs of 'collecting' veins (each pair having right and left veins): the internal iliac veins (IIV), the ovarian veins (OV) and the superior rectal veins (SRV).

The IIV drains 4 groups of afferent tributaries:
1. Anterior visceral veins (uterine, vaginal, vesical and rectal)
2. Parietal veins (inferior gluteal, obturator and pudendal)
3. Posterior pelvic parietal veins (ileolumbar and sacral)
4. Extrapelvic veins (superior gluteal)

There is considerable variability in the drainage of the parietal veins that drain into the anterior branch of the IIV (Figure 1), with 50% draining as a single vein, 36% as a double vein and 14% as a plexiform. The internal iliac vein joins the external iliac vein to form the common iliac vein that combines with the contralateral side to form the inferior vena cava (IVC). On the left the ovarian vein drains (as a single vein in 79%) into the left renal vein (in 99%) or the IVC directly (in 1%). On the right the ovarian vein drains (as a single vein in 78%) into the IVC directly (in 98%) or into the right renal vein (in 2%)[17].

It is important to be aware that there are intra/extra-pelvic anastomoses with the lower limb venous drainage (Figure 2). These can be described as 2 inter-connecting networks: the gluteal-ischiatic venous plexus and the internal pudendal venous plexus[17].

The gluteal vein, draining via the sacral plexus, anastomoses with a collateral from the great saphenous vein (the external circumflex iliac vein), whilst the ischiatic vein, draining the posterior compartment of the thigh, drains into the internal pudendal vein, which itself anastomoses with the femoral vein and great saphenous vein.

The internal pudendal vein anastomoses indirectly with the great saphenous vein via the superficial and deep veins of the clitoris or directly with the external pudendal vein in the labia majora. It is these veins that form vulval varicosities. The internal pudendal vein also forms anastomoses with the perineal tributaries of the anterior visceral veins and the obturator vein.

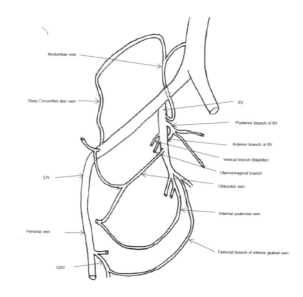

Figure 1: Oblique anatomical view of pelvic venous drainage

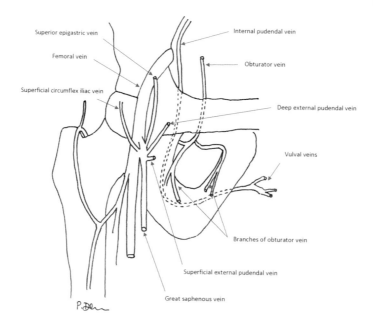

Figure 2: Intra/extra pelvic venous anastomoses with the lower limb and relationship to vulval venous drainage

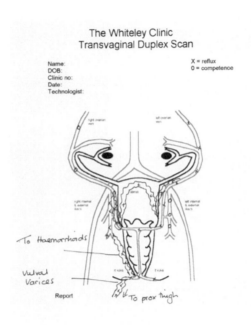

The Whiteley Clinic
Transvaginal Duplex Scan

Name:
DOB:
Clinic no:
Date:
Technologist:

X = reflux
0 = competence

To Haemorrhoids

Vulval
Varices

Report

To prox thigh

Figure 3: Typical TV Duplex scan report

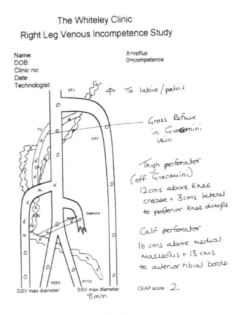

The Whiteley Clinic
Right Leg Venous Incompetence Study

Name:
DOB:
Clinic no:
Date:
Technologist:

X=reflux
0=competence

To labia / pelvis

Gross Reflux
in Giacomini
vein

Thigh perforator
(off Giacomini)
12cms above Knee
crease + 3cms lateral
to posterior Knee dimple

Calf perforator
16 cms above medial
Malleolus + 13 cms
to anterior tibial border

GSV max diameter

SSV max diameter
8mm

CEAP score 2

Figure 4: Typical leg duplex report showing extension of refluxing veins into pelvis

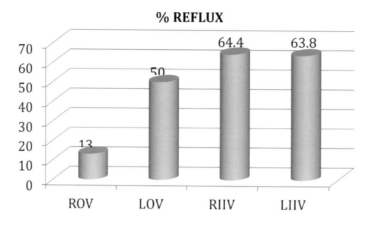

% REFLUX

Figure 5: Distribution of reflux in pelvic veins in an audit of female presenting with leg varicose veins with associated pelvic reflux or symptoms of pelvic congestion syndrome (data kindly supplied by Judith M Holdstock, see Chapter 15).

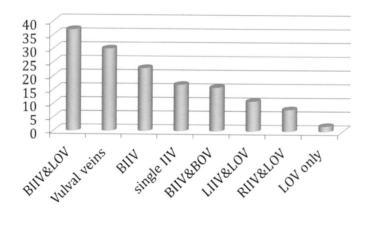

Figure 6: Pattern of reflux in pelvic veins in an audit of female presenting with leg varicose veins with associated pelvic reflux or symptoms of pelvic congestion syndrome (data kindly supplied by Judith M Holdstock, see Chapter 15).

Interpreting the Transvaginal Duplex Scan (TVS)

The TV duplex scan performed pre-operatively is able to identify evidence of flow reversal in the IIV and ovarian vein trunks but it is often difficult to specify exactly which afferent is specifically affected. In considering which veins require embolisation, and subsequently how many coils will be required, it is important to interpret the TVS scan findings in the context of the anatomical clinical presentation of vulval/peri-vulval, buttock or posteromedial thigh varicosities with or without pelvic pain (Figures 3 and 4). The internal pudendal and obturator veins are most closely associated with vulval and posteromedial thigh varicosities. Rich anastomoses are often present between the ovarian veins and these IIV tributaries. The most common pattern of reflux involves both IIV tributaries and the left ovarian vein (Figures 5 and 6).

Endovenous embolisation

Equipment

There are 2 mainstay 5-French guide catheters that are recommended: an angled end-hole catheter, such as a multi-purpose catheter (MPA catheter) and a Simmonds 2 catheter (SIM 2 catheter). A long, stiff hydrophilic guidewire (260cm in length) is recommended for use with the guide catheters. The MPA catheter is used to select the IIV afferent tributaries and the SIM2 the ovarian/gonadal vein. The catheters are introduced via 5-French vascular access sheaths placed in the right internal jugular vein. Iodinated contrast is used to perform the venograms. The procedure can be easily performed with most modern fluoroscopic X-ray C-arms.

Approach

There are 2 approaches that are possible, the femoral or jugular approach. The choice is operator dependant, though the jugular approach has clear advantages in terms of ease of access of the pelvic tributaries and haemostasis post-operatively. An ultrasound guided venous puncture is performed using the Seldinger technique.

Conscious sedation is mostly not required and the procedure may be carried out following local anaesthetic infiltration around the jugular vein puncture alone. Once a 5-French vascular sheath has been placed in the jugular vein, an angled catheter, such as a 5-French multi-purpose (MPA) catheter and 0.035-inch hydrophilic wire, is used to negotiate along the superior vena cava, through the diaphragmatic caval opening and into the inferior vena cava, under fluoroscopic x-ray guidance. In some cases it may be helpful to ask the patient to hold their breath to aid passage of the catheter across the right side of the heart.

Once at the IVC/Iliac confluence the angled catheter and wire are passed into the common and then internal iliac vein. If both internal iliac vein tributaries require intervention, then it is entirely operator choice as to which side is selected first. Once the catheter is placed in the anterior branch of the IIV, venography is used to delineate the afferent tributaries of the IIV (Figure 7). As previously mentioned, there is considerable variability to the pelvic venous anatomy and the venogram provides a "roadmap" by which the relevant afferents can be super-selected.

It is extremely important that, in particular, the internal pudendal and obturator veins and their relevant collaterals are super-selected, given the rich network of intra/extra pelvic anastomoses with the lower limb venous drainage and vulval veins. Despite the variability in appearances of the pelvic venous drainage, the internal pudendal vein and obturator vein can be easily identified and super-selected as the vulval venous drainage is via the internal pudendal vein and the perineal and the leg venous drainage is via the superficial and deep external pudendal vein into the obturator vein tributaries.

Embolisation Material

Once super-selected, it is this author's preference to inject 4-8mls of 3% sodium tetradecyl sulphate foam (Fibrovein) into the internal pudendal and obturator venous tributaries whilst the patient performs the Valsalva manoeuvre. Intra-procedural transvaginal duplex scanning has demonstrated that the Valsalva manoeuvre ensures that foam is drawn into the smaller afferent venous tributaries. This ensures that the smaller afferents inaccessible to the guide catheter are adequately treated. It is unwise to place coils very distally in the vulval veins as patients subsequently have reported that they can often 'feel' the coils when placed as such. Without foam sclerotherapy, there is a greater risk of incomplete obliteration of reflux leading to a potential increased risk of clinical recurrence. The use of foam sclerotherapy, in this setting, also theoretically reduces the risk of pelvic thrombophlebitis. The target afferents are opacified on venography and the foam, made using the Whiteley/Patel method[18], is injected until the contrast is cleared from the afferents, thus ensuring that the target tributaries are satisfactorily filled with foam sclerosant.

Patients often describe a 'stinging' sensation on injection of foam into the IIV afferents. Specifically, they complain of discomfort in the vulva/vagina when the internal pudendal veins are injected and buttock/hip discomfort when the obturator veins are injected. The sensation generally last only a few minutes.

Foam sclerosant is often not required in the ovarian veins, particularly if satisfactory embolisation is achieved of the IIV afferents. Sclerotherapy in the gonadal veins is associated with deep pelvic discomfort on injection. The exception to this is when the IIV afferents are richly anastomosed with a duplex or plexiform ovarian venous drainage.

The use of foam sclerosant is supplemented by the use of fibred endovascular embolisation coils. It is advisable, though not mandatory, to use detachable coils, as these can be repositioned where necessary to ensure accurate placement and retrieved easily if malpositioned. It is difficult to predict exactly how many coils are required to achieve satisfactory embolisation. It is important to size the coil diameter to the average size of the target vein. In general, the minimum size coil selected is 10mm in diameter, with the most common size 12mm (Figure 8). For megalic veins a 15mm coil may be required. The first coil deployed should be 'packed' tightly to form a 'plug'. Subsequent coils can then be deployed whilst withdrawing the guide catheter gradually, to ensure the length of the target vein is covered. It is wise to have a selection of coil lengths (200-400mm) to allow for some flexibility during embolisation. Care must be taken to avoid placement of coils within the IIV trunk, and to restrict placement of coils to the anterior branch of the IIV (Figure 7-12).

Completion of procedure

Unless intra-operative transvaginal duplex is employed, occlusion of the target vein and subsequent non-opacification of the distal vessel is the most reliable end-point for embolisation before termination of the procedure. If the right internal jugular vein approach has been used, once the guide catheter and wire have been withdrawn the vascular sheath can be removed with the patient sat upright at 45° whilst applying manual compression on the puncture site.

172

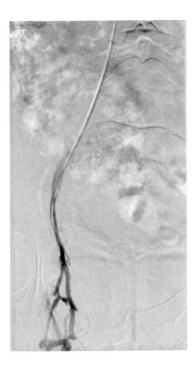

Figure 7: Venogram demonstrating opacification of the obturator vein and its tributaries

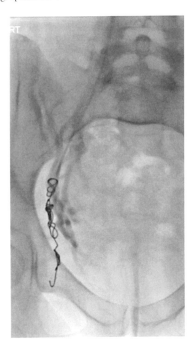

Figure 8: Venogram in the same patient as Figure 7, demonstrating no opacification of the afferent tributaries of the obturator vein following administration of foam sclerosant and deployment of a 12mm x 400mm fibred embolisation coil (Boston Scientific, Massachusetts, USA)

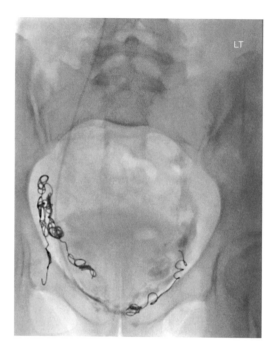

Figure 9: Venogram in same patient demonstrating opacification of the right internal pudendal vein and coils within the left internal pudendal, right obturator and right parauterine veins.

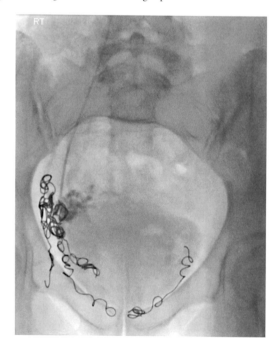

Figure 10: Venogram demonstrating appropriate coil placement (Boston Scientific, Massachusetts, USA) in the internal pudendal veins bilaterally, the right obturator vein and the right parauterine vein. On the right there is opacification of a clump of varices distal to the coils.

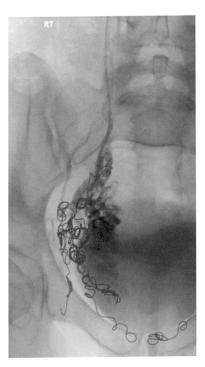

Figure 11: Venogram from the right ovarian vein demonstrates that the previously identified varices close to the anterior branch of the IIV had rich anastomoses with the right ovarian vein.

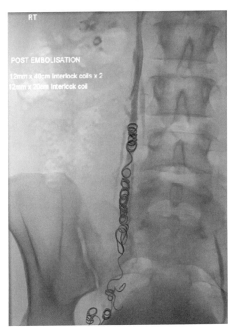

Figure 12: Completion venography demonstrating appropriate deployment of coils (Boston Scientific, Massachusetts, USA) in the right ovarian vein.

Patients are usually recovered in a reclining chair for at least 30 minutes post-procedure before being discharged home the same day. On discharge, it is advisable that the patient is provided with written and verbal post-operative instructions, and that they are advised to return to the clinic in 6-8 weeks for a follow-up transvaginal duplex scan to assess the efficacy of the embolisation and to exclude any new reflux.

Complications of Embolisation

Complications of embolisation of the pelvic veins are rare.

Coil embolisation to the pulmonary circulation with successful retrieval has been reported in the literature[19], though these cases were generally reported in the early experience of the procedure and related to placement of the coils within the main IIV trunk[11], rather than restricting coil placement to refluxing tributaries. When embolisation to the pulmonary artery occurs, it may present as shortness of breath and chest pain immediately after the procedure, or in some cases may be asymptomatic[11]. When symptomatic, it is advisable to remove the coil with the use of an endovascular snare, which can be negotiated into the pulmonary artery via the femoral vein under fluoroscopic guidance.

Inadvertent migration of the coils into the deep common femoral vein has also been reported[11], though with careful deployment at the time of the procedure and use of detachable coils this can be avoided.

There have been reported cases of symptomatic perineal thrombophlebitis[11], though use of intra-operative foam sclerotherapy in the IIV afferents appears to avoid this.

The most common complication following pelvic vein embolisation is post-embolisation syndrome. This is described as transient pyrexia, general aching, gluteal and lumbar pain[20]. The occurrence of this is highly unpredictable and variable. It is self-limiting and is largely controlled by oral Paracetamol and non-steroidal anti-inflammatory medication, such as Ibuprofen.

The majority of patients are fit, healthy and have often never had any medical or surgical history of note previously. Understandably, many have intense procedural related anxiety prior to the procedure. Post-operatively, many of these patients complain of feeling extremely tired and fatigued. Though not widely recognised within the medical literature, this may be due to 'adrenal fatigue', that is thought to be caused by the adrenal glands tiring and subsequently mounting an inadequate response to the level of intense stress. In all cases these symptoms are self-limiting and have resolved by 5-7 days post-procedure.

It is rare for patients to have an allergic reaction to the intravenous x-ray contrast dye used during the procedure, but it is nonetheless advisable to have steroids, adrenaline and anti-histamines available. There has also been a reported case of symptomatic bradycardia, in a case performed under local anaesthetic only, that resolved by administration of atropine[21].

Tips & Tricks and Complex Cases

It is highly recommended that those considering performing PVE familiarise themselves with the wide anatomical variability of pelvic venous drainage. Most of the challenges faced during PVE are due to this wide variation[22].

Complex cases can include apparent absence of the left internal iliac vein with a duplicated IVC, anomalous origin of the anterior division of the IIV arising from the IVC with the posterior division arising from the CIV and the right IIV arising from the left CIV.

Care should be taken to carefully interrogate the CIV for accessory afferents from the internal pudendal or obturator veins draining directly into the EIV or CIV or in some cases the IVC directly.

It is not uncommon for the afferent veins to go into spasm during cannulation. This can be mostly avoided if care is taken when probing the afferent veins and avoiding advancing the catheter without first leading with the guide wire. If, however, spasm does occur then it is best to leave that vein territory and leave at least 15 minutes before attempting again. In some cases the draining afferents may have a scarred and atrophic drainage into the IIV trunk. In these cases, and in other cases where cannulation may be challenging, it may be possible to access the contralateral afferents via the ipsilateral afferents across the midline. Where this is not possible the use of a coaxial microcatheter may be required. Another possible solution to challenging cannulation would be to increase the volume of foam sclerosant with the aim of injecting sclerosant across the midline into the contralateral afferents.

Key learning points
• Have a high index of suspicion of PVI in patients who present with atypical superficial venous reflux and varicose veins, recurrent varicose veins or pelvic pain with no other cause.
• Transvaginal duplex scanning using the Holdstock/Harrison protocol (see Chapter 15) is the gold standard for diagnosis[23] as it can provide
    o   Anatomical information of which vein territories are affected.
    o   Dynamic demonstrable evidence of reflux.
• A detailed understanding of the variability of pelvic venous drainage and the rich anastomoses that exist between the afferent veins is vital in order to correlate the transvaginal duplex scan results with the venogram findings.
• A right jugular approach under local anaesthetic is recommended, using an MPA and SIM 2 catheters over a stiff hydrophilic wire to select the refluxing pelvic and gonadal veins.
• In the deep IIV afferents it is advisable to inject sclerosant foam prior to deploying platinum embolisation coils to ensure effective obliteration of reflux in the small afferents
• Complications are rare and can be mostly avoided by a careful approach.
• Post-embolisation Syndrome and post procedural fatigue is common and unpredictable but self-limiting.

References
1. Perrin MR, Guex JJ, Ruckley CV et al. Recurrent varices after surgery (REVAS): a consensus document. Cardiovasc Surg. 2000; 8(4) :233–45
2. Jones L, Braithwaite BD, Selwyn D et al. Neovascularization is the principal cause of varicose vein recurrence: results of a randomized trial of stripping the long saphenous vein. Eur J

Endovasc Surg. 1996; 12: 442–445

3. Fischer R, Linde N, Duff C et al. Late recurrent sapheno femoral junction reflux after ligation and stripping the greater saphenous vein. J Vasc Surg. 2001; 34: 236–240

4. Hobbs JT. Varicose veins arising from the pelvis due to ovarian vein incompetence. Int J Clin Pract. 2005; 59:1195–1203

5. Labropoulos N, Touloupakis E, Giannoukas AD et al. Recurrent varicose veins: investigation of the pattern and extent of reflux with color flow duplex scanning. Surgery. 1996; 119:406–409

6. Perrin MR, Labropoulos N, Leon LR Jr. Presentation of the patient with recurrent varices after surgery (REVAS). J Vasc Surg. 2006; 43(2):327–334

7. Robinson JC. Chronic pelvic pain. Curr Opin Obstet Gynecol. 1993;5:740-3.

8. Jamieson D, Steege J. The prevalence of dysmenorrhea, dyspareunia, pelvic pain, and irritable bowel syndrome in primary care practices. Obstet Gynecol. 1996;87:55–8.

9. Richet MA. Traite practique d'anatomie medico-chirurgicale. Paris: E Chemeror, Libraire Editeur; 1857.

10. Taylor HC. Vascular congestion and hyperemia; their effects on structure and function in the female reproductive system. Am J Obstet Gynecol. 1949;57:637–53.

11. Ratnam LA, Marsh P, Holdstock JM, Harrison CS, Hussain FF, Whiteley MS, Lopez A. Pelvic Vein Embolisation in the Management of Varicose Veins. Cardiovasc Intervent Radiol. 2008; 31: 1159-1164.

12. Ganeshan A, Upponi S, Hon LQ, Uthappa MC, Warakaulle DR, Uberoi R. Chronic pelvic pain due to pelvic congestion syndrome: the role of diagnostic and interventional radiology. Cardiovasc Intervent Radiol. 2007;30(6):1105–11.

13. Stones RW. Pelvic vascular congestion – half a century later. Clin Obstet Gynecol. 2003;46:831–6.

14. Giacchetto C, Catizone F, Cotroneo GB, et al. Radiologic anatomy of the genital venous system in female patients with varicocele. Surg Gynecol Obstet. 1989;169:403–7.

15. Lefevre H. Broad ligament varicocele. Acta Obstet Gynecol Scand. 1964; 41:122–3.

16. Scultetus AH, Villavicencio JL, Gillespie DL. The nutcracker syndrome: its role in the pelvic venous disorders. J Vasc Surg. 2001;34:812–9.

17. Balian E, Lasry JL, Coppé G, Borie H, Leroux A, Bryon D, Kovarsky S. Pelviperineal venous insufficiency and varicose veins of the lower limbs. Phlebolymphology. 2008;15(1):17-26.

18. Whiteley MS, Patel SB. Modified Tessari Tourbillon technique for making foam sclerotherapy with silicone-free syringes. Phlebology. 2015 Oct; 30: 614-7.

19. Venbrux AC, Chang AH, Kim HS et al. Pelvic congestion syndrome (pelvic venous incompetence): impact of ovarian and internal iliac vein embolotherapy on menstrual cycle and chronic pelvic pain. J Vasc Interv Radiol. 2002; 13:171–178

20. Monedero JL, Ezpeleta SZ, Castro JC et al. Embolization treatment of recurrent varices of pelvic origin. Phlebology. 2006; 21: 3–11

21. Whiteley MS, Lewis-Shiell C, Bishop SI, et. al. Pelvic vein embolisation of gonadal and internal iliac veins can be performed safely and with good technical results in an ambulatory vein clinic, under local anaesthetic alone - Results from two years' experience. Phlebology. 2017 doi: 10.1177/0268355517734952. [Epub ahead of print]

22. Beckett D, Dos Santos SJ, Dabbs EB, Shiangoli I, Price BA, Whiteley MS. Anatomical abnormalities of the pelvic venous system and their implications for endovascular management of pelvic venous reflux. Phlebology 2017 DOI: 10.1177/0268355517735727. [Epub ahead of print]

23. Whiteley M, Dos Santos S, Harrison C, Holdstock J, Lopez A. Transvaginal duplex ultrasonography appears to be the gold standard investigation for the haemodynamic evaluation of pelvic venous reflux in the ovarian and internal iliac veins in women. Phlebology. 2015 Dec; 30: 706-13.

Chapter 17

Healing venous leg ulcers – the role of endovenous surgery to treat superficial venous and perforator vein reflux

Author(s)
Charlotte A Thomas[1,2]
Mark S Whiteley[1,3]

Institution(s)
(1) The Whiteley Clinic, Stirling House, Stirling Road, Guildford, Surrey GU2 7RF
(2) School of Medicine, University of Southampton, UK
(3) Faculty of Health and Biomedical Sciences, University of Surrey, Guildford, Surrey GU2 7XH

Introduction

Venous leg ulcers are a significant health problem in the UK, with an annual incidence of 3.5 per 1000 individuals[1]. They are a severe manifestation of chronic venous insufficiency and are estimated to affect 1% of the adult population with 0.3% of people having an open ulcer at any particular point in time[1-4]. It is estimated that the average yearly cost to treat one venous leg ulcer in the UK is between £546 - £1,338[5]. Furthermore, they are also associated with many health related quality of life issues including pain, malodour, itching, altered appearance and loss of sleep[6]. Prevalence of venous leg ulcers increases with age[7] and the cost of treating patients with venous ulceration is already at least £168 - £198 million per year to the National Health Service[7]. As the world population is growing, the number of people over 60 is expected to double from almost 810 million in 2012 to two billion in 2050[8]. Logically more older people will mean more ulcers and hence, this suggests a significantly increased financial burden on society in the future.

Linton[9] classified the veins of the lower extremity into three systems, deep, superficial and communicating veins which join the deep and superficial systems. He saw that these communicating veins, now referred to as perforators, have valves which only permit blood to move from the superficial into the deep system. His paper highlighted that the valves of the communicating veins become incompetent in the post thrombotic state, noting that incompetence is common in communicating veins just above the medial malleolus. As this also happens to be the most common site of chronic venous ulceration, he suggested an association. Cockett also described the location of the perforating veins just below the calf muscle pump. He highlighted that if valvular incompetence occurs in the perforating veins, a great rise in pressure would be transmitted to the delicate superficial venous mesh on each calf contraction, which could lead to varicose ulcers[10, 11].

In 1938 Linton[12] recommended a treatment for patients suffering with venous leg ulcers. His treatment involved the ligation of the incompetent perforating veins at their origin, beneath the deep fascia. This was achieved via 3 long incisions down the leg; medial, anterolateral and posterolateral. Linton also stated that this should be combined with ligation of the saphenous veins if they were incompetent. In his 1953 paper he gave ulcer recurrence rates of 55% following ligation of communicating veins[9]. The procedure was later modified by Frank Cockett[11], who used a single, medial incision. However, wound complications following open perforator ligation were high, ranging from 12-53%[13]. Cockett found necrosis of the skin edges of the incision occurred in one-fifth of his cases, with rare complications including sepsis and post-operative calf thrombosis[11]. Other complications included infection and wound breakdown that occurred due to the long incision made over unhealthy skin, often leading to prolonged hospitalisation of these patients[13].

Venous hypertension v inflammation

It is still widely believed that venous hypertension is the cause of venous leg ulcers. This theory suggests that high venous pressure in the lower limb leads to damage and skin breakdown forming an ulcer[14]. However, if we consider two people of the same standing height, one with normal veins and valves and one with a venous leg ulcer and complete Great Saphenous Vein (GSV) reflux (i.e. none of the valves in the GSV are working allowing reflux from the right atrium to the ankle), then venous pressure at rest, whether lying down or standing, will be the same in both subjects. The difference between the two clinical scenarios of normal skin or leg ulcer occurs in how this pressure at the ankle, caused by the filling up of the column of blood in the veins, accumulates. In a patient with competent valves, on standing the blood is unable to reflux down the leg from the right atrium and so pressure builds slowly as blood fills into the veins from the arterial system via capillaries. In the patient with venous leg ulcer and GSV reflux, as soon as they stand the blood refluxes immediately all of the way down to the ankle causing an impact pressure and inflammation. Hence it is the rate of change of pressure, not simple venous hypertension, which causes the damage in superficial venous reflux disease (Figures 1 and 2) in mobile patients[15].

The sudden increase in pressure and volume in veins in the ankle acutely stretches the walls and causes inflammation. Smaller veins, venules and capillaries feed these large veins, so the refluxing blood flowing backwards has the same effect on them. The walls of capillaries are only one cell thick and so they are vulnerable to leaking. If there is a leak in the wall, intravascular contents can leak into the tissues and because they contain enzymes and inflammatory mediators an inflammatory response occurs. Over many years as reflux worsens and the veins dilate, the inflammation will cause damage sufficient to affect subcutaneous tissues, dermis and can eventually lead to skin breakdown and leg ulcers[15].

There may be a different mechanism at work in immobile patients with true stasis ulcers who move their leg infrequently, or those with fused ankle joints or other impairments to their leg venous

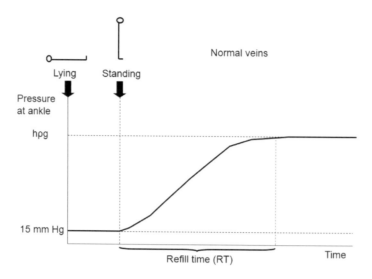

Figure 1: Graphical representation of change of hydrostatic venous pressure at ankle when standing up, in a subject with normal valves in deep and superficial leg veins (from "Understanding Venous Reflux – The cause of varicose veins and venous leg ulcers" Mark S Whiteley)

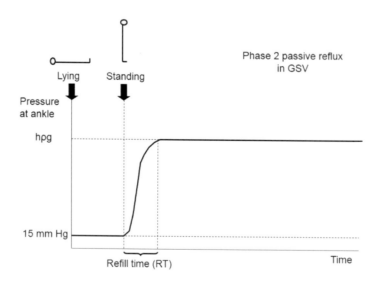

Figure 2: Graphical representation of change of hydrostatic venous pressure at ankle when standing up, in a subject with superficial venous reflux – the final venous pressure at the ankle is the same, but the time to getting to that pressure is very much less (from "Understanding Venous Reflux – The cause of varicose veins and venous leg ulcers" Mark S Whiteley)

pumps. However, this chapter is concerned only with those patients with venous leg ulceration predominantly due to superficial venous reflux, which not only constitutes approximately half of the cases but also are those most easily cured.

With the advent of Duplex Ultrasound in the 1980's, Darke[16] illustrated that 40% of patients with venous leg ulcers had superficial venous incompetence and/or ankle perforating veins, with no reflux in the deep venous system. A further study by Darke[17] showed that 90% of these patients healed with saphenous ligation alone.

More recent studies, suggest that as many as 60% of venous leg ulcers are a result of superficial venous reflux alone[18-20]. Logically these ulcers of venous aetiology are potentially curable with superficial venous surgery.

Venous surgery for venous leg ulcers

In 1999 Professor London showed that by performing open superficial venous surgery alone on patients with venous ulceration and isolated superficial venous incompetence, the large majority could achieve healing, without requiring postoperative compression bandaging, skin grafting or perforator surgery. The study found that at 6, 12 and 18 months healing rates were 57, 74 and 82 per cent respectively[21].

Subfascial endoscopic perforator surgery (SEPS) was the first minimally invasive procedure for leg ulcers and was first introduced in Europe in the mid-1980s by Hauer[22] and Fischer[23]. This technique used a single scope for viewing and working, perforating veins were either clipped or divided or electrocauterised[13]. In 1998 a study[24] found the SEPS procedure led to clinical improvement in 54 out of 57 patients with active or healed ulcerations, with 49% of patients being asymptomatic at follow up (average follow up 17 months).

In 1998, thermoablation of the Great Saphenous Vein using radiofrequency was introduced followed by endovenous laser ablation. These endovenous thermoablation techniques have been shown to be at least as effective as traditional open surgery in the treatment of venous reflux[25-28]. They are now recommended as first line treatment for treating varicose veins[29]. In 2002, our group first described TRansLuminal Occlusion of Perforators (TRLOP), an endovenous version of SEPS[30]. TRLOP is ultrasound guided and only requires a pin-hole skin puncture for cannulation of the incompetent perforator, for passage of the thermoablation device (radiofrequency, laser or other)[31]. We have shown TRLOP to have and equivalent success rate to SEPS in closing incompetent perforating veins even after 5 years[32]. Studies have shown that endovenous techniques can be used to heal venous leg ulcers[33, 34].

A Brazilian group[33] compared EVLA alone against compression therapy in patients with active leg ulcers (CEAP:C6). This concluded that EVLA is safe in patients with active ulcers, importantly finding that in the group treated with EVLA, 81.5% of ulcers had healed at one year follow up compared to 24% in the compression. A cohort study[34] looked at the healing rates of active leg ulcers after treatment with RFA and found that 80% healed without recurrence over the 2.5 year study period.

Compared to open surgery, it is reported that after endovenous surgery patients have less pain, fewer complications, shorter duration of disability, faster return to work and normal activities and a better quality of life[35-39]. There is also evidence emerging that long term recurrence rates of venous reflux with endovenous procedures compared to vein stripping are low. A 10 year follow up of radiofrequency ablation (RFA) procedures in our unit had a successful closure rate of 93.5%[40]. Another study carried out in our unit explored the incidence of revascularisation of the Great Saphenous Vein (GSV) after stripping, it found that at one year revascularisation of the strip-tract occurred in 23% of legs, and in 5% this revascularisation was complete, with the whole length of stripped vein re-growing without valves[41]. Rates of recurrent reflux following traditional surgery are high[36, 42].

In 2011 we performed a retrospective study to look at the healing rate of venous leg ulcers following venous reflux surgery in our unit[43]. It showed our experience of patients who presented with active venous leg ulcers (C6). The patients in our study had previously presented to their local leg ulcer services and had been deemed unfit for surgical treatment, only being offered conservative treatment such as compression bandaging and leg elevation. They arrived at our clinic in search of a second opinion.

The study focused on patients with leg ulcers due to venous reflux, which was reversible using the latest surgical techniques i.e.: superficial or perforator vein reflux. We looked at patients treated between 1999 and 2011 and due to the length of the study period, the surgical techniques used changed significantly. However all treatments aimed to eliminate all superficial venous reflux, truncal and perforator, using the optimal technique available at the time of treatment.

Patients were identified using our computer records and were contacted by letter, telephone or email, inviting them to complete a short questionnaire on the current state of the leg that we had treated. This included 72 patients and, as per our protocol, all of these patients had had their lower

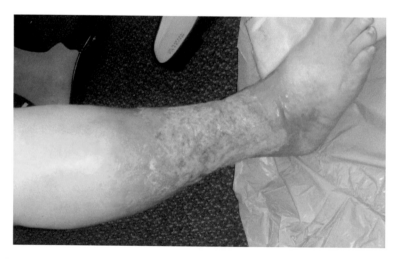

Figure 3: Chronic leg ulcer in lady who had been told she was "incurable" and who had only been given compression bandaging for years. Duplex showed gross reflux in her great saphenous vein (GSV) which was dilated to 20 mm diameter.

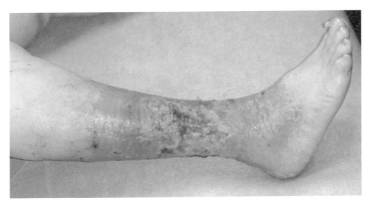

Figure 4: Same lady as in Figure 3. Three weeks post endovenous laser ablation of GSV under local anaesthetic tumescence only and no compression subsequently.

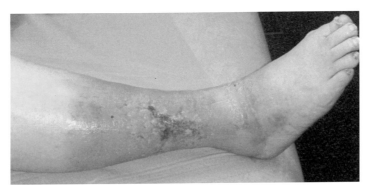

Figure 5: Same lady as in Figure 3. Four weeks post endovenous laser ablation of GSV under local anaesthetic tumescence only and no compression subsequently.

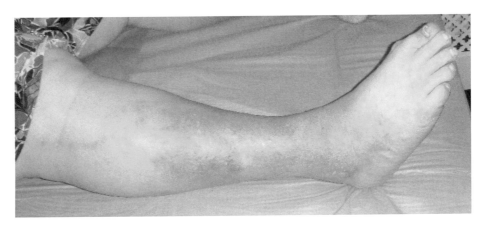

Figure 6: Same lady as in Figure 3. Eight weeks post endovenous laser ablation of GSV under local anaesthetic tumescence only and no compression subsequently.

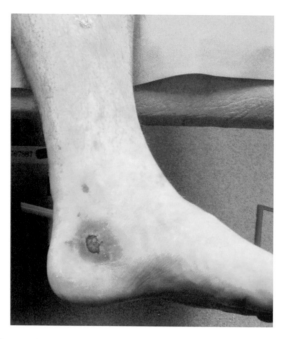

Figure 7: A 19 year old man who had been told that his only treatment option was compression stockings. Duplex ultrasound showed incompetent perforator veins underlying the sub-malleolar ulcer.

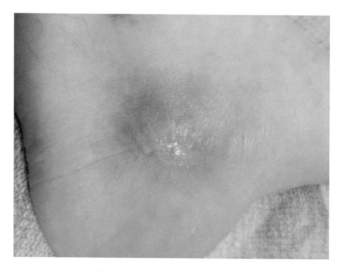

Figure 8: Same patient as in Figure 7, 12 weeks after TRansLuminal Occlusion of Perforators (TRLOP) under local anaesthetic.

limbs scanned using duplex ultrasound to define their reflux patterns prior to their surgery. In the early years, open surgery such as vein stripping and subfascial endoscopic perforator surgery (SEPS) was common practice in our unit. However, as thermoablative therapies developed, techniques such as endovenous laser ablation (EVLA) and radiofrequency ablation (RFA) superseded open surgery.

Fifty patients who had had active ulcers replied to our questionnaire. From the responses, 85% of ulcers had healed, with 52% no longer being confined to any form of long term compression therapy group (see example case in Figures 3 - 8).

We observed that of the 8 ulcers that did not heal with venous surgery, 6 had significant lymphoedema that was severe enough to require preoperative treatment. In ulcers that did heal, 12 of 44 had lymphoedema. This difference was statistically significant ($X2 = 5.76$; $p=0.016$). Lymphoedema has long been recognised as a contributing if not causal factor of leg ulcers, in his 1955 paper, Cockett describes using pre-operative massages and bandaging in order to reduce oedema before operating on incompetent perforating veins[11].

Our study highlighted that there are a large number of patients who are receiving treatment of a conservative nature, i.e. compression bandaging, but are not being offered curative surgery to the underlying cause of their leg ulcers. This leads us to suggest that a more aggressive approach to the investigation and treatment of leg ulcers is required to reduce the number of people suffering with chronic venous leg ulcers. It would also help reduce the burden of wound care on overstretched community and hospital services.

Venous leg ulcers heal faster when using compression therapy than without[44] and the Effect of Surgery and Compression on Healing and Recurrence (ESCHAR)[3] study found no significant difference in healing rate and healing time between superficial venous surgery plus compression and compression alone. However, the advantage of quicker healing post- surgery was hidden by the study design as the time to healing was measured from the start of treatment in the compression arm, but included the wait for surgery in the treatment arm. The study also found that recurrence rates at four years, in patients with isolated superficial reflux, was significantly lower ($p<0.01$) in patients treated with surgery and compression (27%) than in patients treated with compression bandaging alone (51%). This study concluded that 85% of patients with chronic venous leg ulcers would benefit from surgery. As a result of this study, Wright suggested that superficial venous surgery should be considered in all patients with leg ulcers, not to accelerate healing but to prevent recurrence in the future[45].

Costs of leg ulcers to the country

The cost of wound care is significant. A study[46] found that between 2006 and 2007, the cost of wound care was 2.03 million GBP per 100,000 population, requiring 1.44% of the local health-care budget. The main costs included money spent on acute hospital beds, nurses and dressings. In this study leg ulcers represented 28% of wounds, so it is clear that if we can heal leg ulcers more effectively by lowering recurrence with surgery, then a cost saving advantage is to be expected.

References

1.   Simka M, Majewski E. The social and economic burden of venous leg ulcers: focus on the role of micronized purified flavonoid fraction adjuvant therapy. Am J Clin Dermatol.

2003;4(8):573-81.

2. Abbade LPF, Lastoria S. Venous ulcer: epidemiology, physiopathology, diagnosis and treatment. Int J Dermatol. 2005;44:449–56

3. Barwell JR, Davies CE, Deacon J, Harvey K, Minor J, Sassano A, et al. Comparison of surgery and compression with compression alone in chronic venous ulceration (ESCHAR study): randomised controlled trial. Lancet. 2004;363:1854-9.

4. Bradbury AW. Epidemiology and aetiology of C4-6 disease. Phlebology. 2010;25:2–8

5. Ragnarson Tennvall G, Hjelmgren J. Annual costs of treatment for venous leg ulcers in Sweden and the United Kingdom. Wound Repair Regen. 2005;13(1):13-8

6. Hareendran A, Bradbury A, Budd J et al. Measuring the impact of venous leg ulcers on quality of life. J Wound Care. 2005;14(2):53-7

7. Posnett J, Franks P J. The burden of chronic wounds in the UK. Nursing Times. 2008;104(3):44-5

8. United Nations Population Fund, HelpAge International. Ageing in the Twenty-First Century A Celebration and A Challenge. New York: United Nations Population Fund;2012.

9. Linton RR. The post thrombotic ulceration of the lower extremity: its etiology and surgical treatment. Ann Surg. 1953;138:415-32.

10. Cockett FB. Jones BD. The ankle blow-out syndrome: a new approach to the varicose ulcer problem. Lancet. 1953;i:17-23

11. Cockett FB. The pathology and treatment of venous ulcers of the leg. Br J Surg. 1955;43:260-78.

12. Linton RR. The operative treatment of varicose veins and ulcers, based upon a classification of these lesions. Ann Surg. 1938; 107: 582–93.

13. Rhodes JM, Gloviczki P. Surgery of Perforating veins, In: Ballard JL, Bergan JJ (eds), Chronic Venous Insufficiency, Diagnosis and Treatment. London: Springer; 2000. p103-116.

14. NHS Choices. Leg Ulcer, venous. http://www.nhs.uk/conditions/Leg-ulcer-venous/Pages/Introduction.aspx

15. Whiteley MS. Understanding venous reflux - The cause of varicose veins and venous leg ulcers. Milton Keynes UK: Whiteley Publishing Limited; 2011.

16. Sethia KK, Darke SG. Long saphenous incompetence as a cause of venous ulceration. Br J Surg. 1984;71:754–5

17. Darke SG, Penfold C. Venous ulceration and saphenous ligation. Eur J Vasc Surg. 1992;6:4–9

18. Shami SK, Sarin S, Cheatle TR, Scurr JH, Smith PD. Venous ulcers and the superficial venous system. J Vasc Surg. 1993;17:487–90

19. Bergqvist D, Lindholm C, Nelze´n O. Chronic leg ulcers: the impact of venous disease. J Vasc Surg. 1999;29:752–5

20. Scriven JM, Hartstone T, Bell PRF, Naylor AR, London NJM. Single-visit venous ulcer assessment clinic: the first year. Br J Surg. 1997;84:334–6

21. Bello M, Scriven M, Hartshorne T, Bell PRF, Naylor AR, London NJM. Role of superficial venous surgery in the treatment of venous ulceration. Br J Surg. 1999;86:755–9

22. Hauer G. Endoscopic subfascial discussion of perforating veins—preliminary report. (In German.) Vasa. 1985; 14: 59–61.

23. Fischer R. Experience with endoscopic perforator interruption. (In German.) Phlebologie. 1992; 21: 224–29.

24. Rhodes JM, Gloviczki P, Canton LG, Rooke T, Lewis BD, Lindsey JR. Factors affecting clinical outcome following endoscopic perforator vein ablation. Am J Surg. 1998; 176: 162–67.20.

25. Nesbitt C, Eifell RKG, Coyne P, Badri H, Bhattacharya V,Stansby G. Endovenous ablation (radiofrequency and laser) and foam sclerotherapy versus conventional surgery for great saphenous vein varices. Cochrane Database of Systematic Reviews. 2011;(10):CD005624. DOI: 10.1002/14651858.CD005624.pub2

26. Dindyal S, Woddburn KR. Changing practice from conventional surgery to endovenous treatments produces excellent results for both long and short saphenous varicose veins. Ann R Coll Surg Engl. 2010;92:85-90

27. Hinchcliffe RJ, Ubhi J, Beech A, Ellison J, Braithwaite BD. A Prospective Randomised Controlled Trial of VNUS Closure versus Surgery for the Treatment of Recurrent Long Saphenous Varicose Veins. Eur J Vasc Endovasc Surg. 2006;31:212-8

28. Min RJ, Khilnani N, Zimmet SE. Endovenous Laser Treatment of Saphenous Vein Reflux: Long-Term Results. J Vasc Interv Radiol. 2003;14(8):991-6

29. Varicose veins in the legs. The diagnosis and management of varicose veins. National Institute for Health and Care Excellence. London 2013; CG168.

30. Kianifard B, Browning L, Holdstock J M, Whiteley MS. Surgical technique and preliminary results of perforator vein closure - TRLOPS (Transluminal Occlusion of perforators).Br J Surg. 2002; 89: 507-526.

31. Mark S Whiteley, Judy HoldstockPercutaneous radiofrequency ablations of Varicose Veins (VNUS Closure) In: Roger M Greenhalgh ed, Vascular and Endovascular Challenges . London; BibaPublishing. 2004. p 361- 381

32. Bacon JL, Dinneen AJ, Marsh P, Holdstock JM, Price BA, Whiteley MS. Five-year results of incompetent perforator vein closure using TRans-Luminal Occlusion of Perforator. Phlebology. 2009;24(2):74-8

33. Viarengo LM, Potério-Filho J, Potério GM, Menezes FH, Meirelles GV. Endovenous laser treatment for varicose veins in patients with active ulcers: measurement of intravenous and perivenous temperatures during the procedure. Dermatol Surg. 2007 Oct;33(10):1234-42

34. Marrocco C J, Atkins MD, Bohannon WT, Warren TR, Buckley CJ, Bush RL. Endovenous Ablation for the Treatment of Chronic Venous Insufficiency and Venous Ulcerations. World Journal of Surgery 2010;34(10:)2299-2304

35. Murad H, Coto-Yglesias F, Zumaeta-Garcia M et al. A systematic review and meta-analysis

of the treatments of varicose veins. J Vasc Surg 2011;53(165):49S-65S

36.   Lurie F, Creton D, Eklof B et al. Prospective Randomised Study of Endovenous Radiofrequency Obliteration (closure) Versus Ligation and Vein Stripping (EVOLVeS): Two-year Follow-up. Eur J Vasc Endovasc Surg 2005;29:67-73

37.   Ugur Ozkan, Sariturk C. Early clinical improvement in chronic venous insufficiency symptoms after laser ablation of saphenous veins. Diagn Interv Radiol 2012 Jul (ePub ahead of print)

38.   Vuylsteke M, Van den Bussche D, Audenaert EA, Lissens P. Endovenous laser obliteration for the treatment of primary varicose veins. Phlebology 2006;21:80-87.

39.   McBride KD. Changing to endovenous treatment for varicose veins: How much more evidence is needed? The Surgeon 2011;9(3):150-9

40.   Taylor D, Whiteley A, Fernandez-Hart T, Whiteley M. Ten Year Results of Radiofrequency Ablation (VNUS Closure®) of the Great Saphenous and Anterior Accessory Saphenous Veins in the Treatment of Varicose Veins Tecnicas endovasculares. April 2013;Vol XVI (1):134

41.   Munasinghe A, Smith C, Kianifard B, Price B A, Holdstock J M, Whiteley M S. Strip-track revascularization after stripping of the great saphenous vein. Br J Surg. 2007;94:840–3

42.   Allaf N, Welch M. Recurrent varicose veins: Inadequate surgery remains a problem. Phlebology. 2005;20:138–40

43.   Thomas CA, Holdstock JM, Harrison CC, Price BA, Whiteley MS. Healing rates following venous surgery for chronic venous leg ulcers in an independent specialist vein unit. Phlebology. 2013:28:132–139

44.   O'Meara S, Cullum NA, Nelson EA. Compression for venous leg ulcers (Review). Cochrane Database Syst Rev 2009;(1):CD000265

45.   Wright DD. The ESCHAR trial: should it change practice? Perspect Vasc Surg Endovasc Ther. 2009; 21(2):69-72

46.   Vowden K, Vowden P, Posnett J. The resource costs of wound care in Bradford and Airedale primary care trust in the UK. J Wound Care. 2009 Mar;18(3):93-4, 96-8

Chapter 18

Healing Leg Ulcers by Interventions on Obstructed Deep Veins

Author
Robbie George

Institution
Narayana Institute of Vascular Sciences, Bangalore, India

Introduction
The estimated prevalence of active venous ulcers is 0.8 to 1 per 1000 population[1]. Change and improvements in the delivery and organization of care have improved outcomes but failure to heal and recurrence rates of up to 34% continue to be an expensive problem[1]. The mainstay of leg ulcer management continues to be compression therapy but this is not the subject of this chapter.

Venous leg ulcers are thought to be a consequence of multiple etiologies. Traditionally, the predominant factor in the development of venous ulceration was considered to be reflux secondary to valvular incompetence. However, as demonstrated in the ESCHAR trial, treatment of the superficial venous reflux only reduces ulcer recurrence without having an impact on ulcer healing when compared to compression therapy alone. Other factors such as venous outflow resistance have usually been ignored. The contribution of obstructive pathology in the iliac vein in the development of venous disease has been unrecognized for many years. In the last few decades, seminal work by Raju and Neglen once again brought to attention the contribution of deep venous pathology in the evolution of venous disease.

Anatomy and Etiology
The superficial and deep venous systems of the leg unite at the common femoral vein to drain as the external iliac vein that is joined by the internal iliac vein and other pelvic veins to become the common iliac vein. The common iliac vein confluence lies posterior to the aorta and the iliac arteries - this anatomical location of a low pressure venous system behind the high pressure arterial system has implications for the development of disease.

Within the venous system of the leg, there exist various mechanisms to mitigate the effect that erect posture of the homo-sapiens has on the venous blood pressure in the most dependent portions of the leg. Significant among these systems are the presence of valves, which permit only centripetal flow within the veins. In addition, the calf pump also encourages the maintenance of centripetal flow.

In a certain group of patients the overlying iliac artery compresses the iliac veins. This non-thrombotic iliac vein lesion (NIVL) is commoner on the left side where the proximal common iliac vein compression is caused by the right common iliac artery. This particular anatomical situation of primary Non-thrombotic Iliac Vein Lesion (NIVL) causing obstruction was described originally by McMurrich[2] in 1908 and brought to prominence by May and Thurner[3] in 1957 and is known eponymously as the May-Thurner syndrome, Cockett syndrome or iliac vein compression syndrome.

NIVL is surprisingly common in the general population and autopsy studies have demonstrated intraluminal lesions in 20-30% of cadaveric dissections[3-5]. Iliac vein compression by the artery is common in the general population, even those without any kinds of symptoms[6]. However, this pattern is seen in even greater frequency among patients with chronic venous disease symptoms. These intraluminal lesions may range from simple webs and ridges to complete occlusion[3].

NIVL is a controversial subject, especially its relevance to the development of symptoms. Given how commonly this anatomical appearance exists in the normal population, its clinical significance has been doubted and has even been classed as a normal anatomical variant[7]. Raju and Neglen have proposed that NIVL be viewed as a permissive lesion i.e. it exists silently until another factor is added which triggers a symptomatic clinical presentation[8]. They have likened its existence to a patent foramen ovale presenting with a paradoxical embolus in that there exists a silent pathological lesion that is unveiled only when a further clinical event occurs.

The iliac vein can also be a site of deep vein thrombosis (DVT), either *de novo* or as a consequence of a NIVL. Studies have shown that among patients with CVI with history of DVT an obstructive component predominates in approximately 30% of symptomatic limbs. A combination of reflux and obstruction is observed in over half of the symptomatic population[9,10].

Deep vein thrombosis is the commonest cause of iliac vein obstruction. As the common outflow tract for the limb, any occlusion or stenosis at this level has profound effects on the limb, as adequate collateralization to compensate for a large diameter vein such as the iliac is difficult to achieve. It is known that only 20-30% of iliac veins completely re-canalize after an occlusion and the majority reopen only partially and are compensated for by varying extents of collateralization[10, 11]. Other rare causes of partial or complete obstruction of the deep veins include malignant tumors, iatrogenic injury, retroperitoneal fibrosis, trauma, irradiation, cysts, aneurysms and pelvic masses.

History and Physical Examination

Signs and symptoms of venous hypertension can often be elicited on history and examination. Common among these tend to be itching and dry skin.

A prominent symptom, seen often in the absence of signs, is venous claudication. This is described as a bursting pain in the thigh or leg brought on by exercise and relieved only by rest and limb elevation. The relief of pain typically takes at least 10 minutes, which helps differentiate it from arterial claudication.

A history of DVT should be specifically elicited. A number of patients may have suffered a silent

DVT in the past and a history of limb swelling around the time of surgery, pregnancy or trauma in the presence of venous ulceration should raise suspicions that this could be a post-thrombotic syndrome (PTS) presentation.

Examination may reveal the presence of obvious varicose veins in the lower limbs. Often cross-pubic collaterals may be seen with large saphena varix in the groin. Other signs of chronic venous insufficiency such as lipodermatosclerosis, eczema and pigmentation may be seen.

Classically venous ulcers are indolent sloughy painless ulcers seen typically at the medial malleolus. They tend to be indolent and recurrent even if healed[1]. The ulcers often exist on a background of other skin changes such as lipodermatosclerosis and eczema with pigmentation.

Investigations
A variety of investigations are available to investigate patients with venous disease.

Presently the investigation of choice for detection of venous pathology is Intra Vascular Ultrasound (IVUS). According to clinical users of the system, a significant proportion of venous pathology is missed by other diagnostic modalities.

Thrombophilia workup
Patients with a history suggestive of DVT or those whose imaging suggests that the venous disease is a consequence of a previous undiagnosed DVT should probably undergo a preoperative thrombophilia workup. This should comprise of antithrombin 3, homocystine, protein C and S, anticardiolipin antibody, lupus anticoagulant, prothrombin and Leiden gene mutation screening.

The presence of an underlying thrombophilic condition has implications for the postoperative management.

Venous Doppler
The first line is to obtain an adequate venous duplex to study the deep and superficial systems. There can be clues to an upstream problem on the venous Doppler, such as evidence of deep venous reflux of more than 1 second or unusual dilatation of the common femoral vein especially when compared to the opposite side. In addition, evidence of previous DVT in the form of recanalization and webs is often associated with pathology within the iliac segment as well. In addition the presence of significant venous disease especially in the absence of Saphenofemoral junction or Saphenopopliteal junction reflux should raise a suspicion of upstream disease. Of note in the ESCHAR trial nearly 20% of patients had venous ulcers without evidence of significant reflux in the superficial system[12].

CT and MR Venography
Imaging of the deeper veins in the pelvis and abdomen is often inadequate with Duplex ultrasound. CT has been utilized as a tool to demonstrate thrombosis both in deep veins and pulmonary arteries. Most research has focused on CT identification of DVT, rather than NIVL or post-thrombotic changes.

There are no established techniques or diagnostic criteria for the diagnosis of central vein pathology on CT. Oguzkurt et al.[13] have described their findings in 10 cases. Jeon et al.[14] divided patients with left common iliac vein obstruction into 3 groups: focal compression, atrophy and complete obliteration, which is a practical method of assessing the pathology.

In our practice we often utilize CT Venogram as a tool to select patients for further interventions. Unfortunately the awareness and detection of iliac vein pathology by radiologists appears to be quite poor and we therefore tend to inspect all CT images ourselves. On occasion, the pathology is obvious with an occluded "cord like" iliac vein or IVC seen. There are other more subtle signs we look for as well. These include the presence of abnormal collaterals, a difference in diameter of the iliac veins and visible compression of the iliac veins by overlying arteries. In this context, it is important to recognize that venous compression may occur at sites other than the classic May-Thurner point as is illustrated in Figure 1.

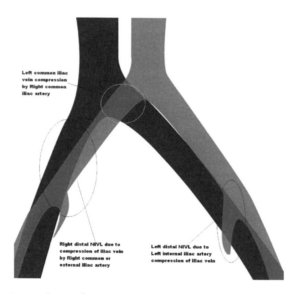

Figure 1: Diagram showing usual sites of venous compression in the iliac veins

We also look for evidence of thrombotic disease within the Femoral and Profunda Femoris veins. Often the Profunda Femoris vein has enlarged and has become the primary deep vein of the leg in the presence of Femoral vein disease. This collateralization has implications for choice of access site if an endovascular intervention is planned. The other benefit of CT is that it is able to detect other abdominal or pelvic pathology that may be the cause of secondary venous reflux.

MR Venogram
MRI has always been attractive, as it does not expose the patient to radiation or iodinated contrast.

Most research in MRV has also been devoted to the identification of DVT. NIVL, pelvic congestion syndromes and other chronic venous diseases have been investigated by some authors and they have shown that adequate imaging of the venous system from calf to IVC is possible with different imaging protocols[15,16,17]. Post thrombotic changes such as webs, trabeculations, fibrosis etc. have been depicted but well defined diagnostic criteria still remain elusive.

IVUS

Intravascular ultrasound is especially popular for the assessment of coronary interventions. Raju and Neglen have been great proponents of IVUS as the gold standard for the diagnosis of venous pathology and have described their technique in detail[11]. They have demonstrated that venous IVUS appears superior to single-plane venography for the morphologic diagnosis and also in guiding stent placement. The technique is especially useful in the detection of subtle intraluminal pathology that is not seen on standard venography.

Essentially the technique involves crossing the area of suspected pathology with a wire, following which the IVUS catheter is tracked on the wire and the venous system interrogated with the help of specialized software. The authors have utilized a 6F, 12.5 MHz imaging catheter (Sonicath Ultra 6, Boston Scientific Corp., Watertown, MA, USA) with the SONOS system (SONOS Intravascular Diagnosis System M2400A, Hewlett Packard, Andover, MA, USA). On IVUS morphologic obstruction of >50% of the luminal diameter has been considered an indication for venous stenting[11].

This has also been supported by the work of others who have demonstrated that other imaging techniques fail to adequately diagnose NIVL[18]. However, the availability of IVUS and peripheral catheters in appropriate sizes for regular use continues to be a problem in many centres, including ours.

Venogram

Venographic features of iliac vein pathology can range from the obvious occlusion with collaterals to subtle findings to a completely normal appearance. Traditionally venography has been performed by injection into foot vessels – this, however, suffers from the poor visualization of pelvic vessels. A transfemoral venogram provides much better visualization of the pelvic veins and also allows the performance of a descending Venogram if primary refluxive pathology is suspected.

Obvious features of disease are venous occlusion with the presence of a large number of pelvic collaterals. More subtle signs include the presence of a small number of collateral vessels with varying appearances of the iliac vein. The vein may show "pancaking" of contrast, or occasionally an impression of extrinsic compression, or a streaky appearance to contrast[10]. The latter is especially seen in patients who have had a DVT which has recanalised in a sieve like fashion. An additional step we often take in our practice is to do a trial balloon dilatation and observe for a waist on the balloon. Balloons appropriate to the vein diameter are used. This method is utilized whenever the venogram appears grossly normal.

Interventions

Iliac vein angioplasty and stenting

Endovascular methods have revolutionized the management of deep vein pathology. The original reports of large series came from Riveroaks[19] and Marseille[20]. The procedure can be safely performed under local anesthesia and often as a day case office procedure. Access is obtained by a femoral puncture in the groin. If the femoral vein or CFV confluence is involved venous access must be obtained more distally in the leg - either the femoral vein in mid-thigh or the popliteal vein or even the small saphenous vein if it is adequately dilated. This access may be obtained blind, guided by anatomical landmarks or under ultrasound guidance.

Once access has been established, Heparin is administered intravenously in a dose of 80 IU/kg.

The first step is to obtain an adequate venogram looking for the signs of venous stenosis or occlusion described earlier. If IVUS is available, it should be utilized to interrogate the venous system.

If the findings are consistent with the need for an intervention, it is important to ensure that the access sheaths are of adequate diameter as often 9 or 10 Fr sizes are required for passage of the large diameter balloons and stents.

Stenting

The lesion is crossed using a combination of a hydrophilic wire and an angled catheter. Crossing a lesion can be a very simple or a very prolonged procedure dependent on its nature. Recanalisation of an occluded iliac vein and IVC can be a tedious procedure but with perseverance most lesions can be crossed. Sometimes it may require a combined approach from a femoral and jugular access. Occasionally the guide wire may perforate the vein wall resulting in contrast extravasation - such bleeding is invariably minor and settles without need for intervention. On occasion when it is impossible to cross the lesion, it may become feasible on another occasion.

Once the lesion is crossed the segment is angioplastied with diameters appropriate to the area. For the IVC we use 20-24 mm balloons, common iliac vein 14-16 mm, external iliac vein 12-14 mm and common femoral vein 10-12 mm. Like most venous angioplasties, this inflation can be quite painful and adequate parenteral analgesia especially while dilating chronic occlusions may be required.

Almost every significant venous lesion will need a stent to keep it open. Unlike the arterial system with its high pressure intraluminal flows and a well-developed tunica media, the venous system has very little incentive to stay open in the presence of a fibrotic or externally compressive lesion. The original work from Riveroaks and Marseille has described extensive use of long stainless steel self-expanding stents - namely the Wallstent™ (Boston Scientific-Schneider, Minneapolis,MN,USA). In our own experience of around 90 limbs we have made extensive use of self-expanding Nitinol stents (ELuminexx™, Bard Corporation etc.). We have found the stents to be robust with excellent radial strength, flexibility and are available in appropriate sizes especially for the iliac system.

Some technical points regarding the technique of stenting are noteworthy.

Firstly, it is essential to stent the entire abnormal area i.e. to go from healthy inflow to healthy outflow. In the common iliac veins this implies that the stent must extend well into the IVC. It is important to recognize that venography significantly underestimates the extent of disease and therefore the stents need to extend generously in both directions. It is important to have a good selection of long length stents available for this purpose - our most commonly used size is the 14 mm x 120 mm long stent.

It is essential to ensure adequate inflow, both to relieve the venous hypertension and to ensure the stents do not thrombose. This is especially relevant where the etiology is post thrombotic. The common femoral vein is often involved in the thrombotic process and stents should be liberally extended into this area. Unlike the arterial system there have never been any reports of stent fracture or complication due to stents crossing the inguinal ligament.

Where required multiple stents may be used. When doing so it is important to ensure that adequate overlap is achieved to avoid any unsupported areas.

Post procedure management

The sheaths are removed shortly after completion of the procedure and the patient may begin to mobilise within a few hours.

The optimal anticoagulation regime is still unknown with differing practices worldwide[21,22,23]. Any patient with a known prothrombotic state should be recommenced on their original anticoagulation regime with appropriate low molecular weight heparin cover. The duration of anticoagulation is determined by the underlying prothrombotic state.

In the absence of a known prothrombotic state our own policy is to commence therapeutic low molecular weight heparin for 5 days and overlap this with Warfarin until an INR of 2 is achieved. The INR is monitored and maintained between 2-3, for the next 3 months. Warfarin is stopped at 3 months and Aspirin 75mg once a day is initiated for life, unless there are other contraindications.

Some units tend not to anticoagulate at all while others will not undertake the procedure unless the patient is anticoagulated preoperatively and the regime continued for 6 months post procedure.

Results and outcomes

Technical success

Technical success of achieving stenting in NIVL and stenotic lesions is 100% but ranges from 67-95% for chronic total occlusions[24,25,26,27,28]. Longer term stent patency is also dictated by the primary pathology. Primary assisted patency among stents placed for NIVL ranges from 42%-100%[21], while 5 year patency for post thrombotic lesions is lower at 58-75%[21,29-32].

Ulcer outcomes

The largest series with longer term follow up of leg ulcers is again from Raju and Neglen[21]. In their report from 2007 they reported outcomes of ulcer healing in 148 limbs followed up for a mean period of 23 months. Ulcer healing was achieved in 101 limbs with recurrence in 8 limbs over the follow up period. The cumulative ulcer healing rate at 5 years was 58% (50% with stent alone and 57% with adjunctive procedures) for patients with NIVL and 55% for thrombotic limbs[21]. Similar results, albeit of smaller series, have been reported by Alhalbouni et al.[25] and Rosales et al.[26]. Our own experience of 40 limbs has shown an ulcer healing rate of 60% at 14 months follow up. The ulcer resolution and symptom relief can be dramatic in some patients with long standing recalcitrant ulcers disappearing in a matter of weeks.

Open surgery

Open surgery has fallen out of favour since the advent of endovascular techniques with its minimum morbidity and good results. Today open reconstruction with venous bypass is reserved for those who fail attempts at stenting or those who are not candidates for endovascular procedures[24,33-35]. The latter group would include cases of iliac vein occlusion secondary to iatrogenic injuries associated with ligation or clipping of the vein, those with associated venous aneurysms or rarely those with infiltrating malignant tumors[24,33-35].

Open surgery may have a role as a hybrid procedure wherein an endovenectomy of the common femoral vein may be combined with stenting in the ilio-caval system[24].

Surgical considerations and procedure

The key factors determining outcome are the quality of inflow and outflow, the conduit utilized and whether there are any underlying prothrombotic conditions.

Inflow and Outflow

As for all endovascular procedures, it is essential to have adequate inflow and non-obstructed outflow for a venous bypass graft to remain patent. Inflow and outflow assessment will need a combination of venous duplex and venography to identify target areas. The inflow will rarely be taken caudal to the femoral level, while the outflow could be the contralateral femoral vein or the infra-hepatic IVC.

Conduit

A variety of conduits are available but all have their problems[36]. There has been a lot of work in the development of large diameter prosthetic conduits and better patencies are now possible but, as in most areas, autologous conduits remain the best[36].

The saphenous vein is a readily available conduit, provided it is of a reasonable size. The contralateral saphenous vein may be utilized for a femoro-femoral bypass provided it is available and not involved in the disease process. The saphenous vein may also be utilized to create a spiral graft, but it does not perform as well[36].

The contralateral femoral vein is a large diameter conduit that can be used. However, the removal of a femoral vein in a patient group that most likely has a significant history of thrombotic disease is not without its own attendant complications.

Autologous cryopreserved femoral vein has been utilized for reconstruction but with relatively poor results[37].

Other potential sources for autologous conduit would include the external or internal jugular veins, basilica vein and its continuation into the brachial and axillary veins.

Among the synthetic conduits the graft of choice would be expanded polytetrafluorethylene (ePTFE)[36,37,39-41]. It is available in a large variety of large diameters and configurations and also with additional external support. The latter feature is very attractive as the venous system has a low pressure and could be easily compressed against the inguinal ligament or secondary to increased intra-abdominal pressure[37].

Adjuncts to improve patency

Arteriovenous fistula

Kunlin in 1953 was the first to describe creation of an adjunctive arteriovenous fistula to improve patency of the venous graft[42]. This has been confirmed by numerous authors[34,43-45]. The arteriovenous fistula increases flows that are thought to reduce platelet and fibrin deposition and hence maintain graft patency[44]. This is probably more significant for synthetic conduits which need a higher flow rate to maintain patency owing to their increased thrombogenecity. The arteriovenous fistula can be constructed using a branch of the saphenous vein and connecting it to the superficial femoral artery[36]. The procedure adds to the operative time and will often need a second surgery for ligation. An arteriovenous fistula may also contribute to venous hypertension by virtue of the increased flows. An additional AV fistula is recommended for prosthetic grafts anastomosed to the femoral vein and for iliocaval grafts longer than 10 cm[36]. The fistula is left running for at least 6 months, and even lifelong if there are no side effects[36].

The surgical procedure may be limited to an endovenectomy of the common femoral vein or may be combined with a bypass procedure[35].

Thrombosis prophylaxis

As a group these patients are very vulnerable to a new thrombotic event and every precaution must be taken to prevent this. Intravenous heparin at a dose of 80 IU/Kg is administered prior to venous clamping and a heparin infusion is commenced to maintain a target aPTT ratio of 1.5 - 2.0 times normal until recovery. Thereafter low molecular weight heparin is started and then converted to Warfarin.

Bypass Configuration

Various configurations of the bypass are possible, dependent upon the anatomy and available conduit.

Popliteal-femoral bypass

Today the classic May-Husni procedure of a popliteal-femoral bypass using saphenous vein with a differential arteriovenous fistula in the calf is rarely performed.

Femoro-femoral bypass

Palma and Esperon[46,47] described the technique of using normal contralateral saphenous vein to bypass the iliac occlusion in a cross-pubic fashion. This procedure requires a normal iliac venous system on the contralateral side to provide drainage. The saphenous vein should be healthy and of at least 4 mm diameter to be considered suitable. We always add a differential arteriovenous fistula to encourage flows and maintain patency. Normally the saphenous vein is only transected at the caudal end and transposed to the opposite femoral vein. If however the angulation is too much, the vein may be divided and re-anastomosed to the femoral vein in a more haemodynamically suitable configuration. If the saphenous vein is not suitable, the same procedure is carried out using a ringed ePTFE graft of 8-10mm diameter with an added arteriovenous fistula.

Femoro-Caval and Ilio-Caval Bypass

The bypass may also be configured as a femoro-caval or ilio-caval bypass. In either case large diameter externally supported ePTFE grafts are preferred. A 10-12 mm graft for a femoro-caval bypass and 14-20mm grafts for more central veins. We and most other authors would add an arteriovenous fistula to the femorocaval bypass.

Outcomes

The worldwide experience of open surgical reconstructions for venous occlusions is very limited. Most series precede the endovascular era, and none report data exclusively for patients with venous ulceration. Halliday et al.[48] and AbuRahma et al.[49] reported 5 year patency of 75% each for patients undergoing the Palma procedure with a vein conduit. The patency for prosthetic bypass of the ilio-caval segment at 20 months was reported at 88% by Alimi et al.[40] and 54% at 2 years by Jost et al.[34].

In 2011 Gloviczki et al. reported on their experience of 60 patients undergoing open or hybrid repairs[24,35]. This is the largest and most recent series to date and included 12 patients with active ulcers and 6 with healed ulcers.

Overall among the 60 patients graft patency was poor with early re-occlusions in 17% after open repairs and 33% after hybrid procedures. A significant number of patients need further interventions to maintain patency.

Five year primary and secondary patency for all procedures has been reported at 43% and 58% respectively. The Palma vein grafts do better with primary and secondary patency reported at 70% and 78% respectively. Femoro-caval bypasses perform relatively poorly with 5-year primary assisted patency of 57%.

Ulcer healing was achieved in 10 of 12 patients at 12 months; the two patients with persistent ulcers had an early graft occlusion that could not be salvaged. Among the 10 who achieved healing 50% recurred at a mean of 48 months after reconstruction. Among this group 3 had a patent bypass.

Summary

Venous ulcers can be a chronic and expensive problem, both for the individual and society. Much attention has been focused on management of the local wound and of the refluxive pathology in the superficial venous system. The contribution of obstruction within the deep veins of the pelvis has largely been ignored. Recent data and experience have shown that a significant number of patients with venous ulcers have undiagnosed iliac vein pathology.

The element of Non-thrombotic Iliac Vein Lesion (NIVL) may exist as a permissive lesion and is seen in greater frequency among the population with venous disease. Most venous lesions are eminently suitable to endovascular interventions in the form of iliac vein angioplasty and stenting. Up to 60% of ulcers can be expected to heal and stay healed. Patients with post thrombotic iliac vein lesions do not fare as well as those with NIVL. Today the indications for open surgery for ilio-caval obstructions are few.

References

1. Callam MJ, Harper DR, Dale JJ, Ruckley CV. Chronic ulcer of the leg: clinical history. Br Med J. 1987; 294: 1389-91.

2. McMurrich JP. The occurrence of congenital adhesions in the common iliac veins and their relation to thrombosis of the femoral and iliac veins. Am J Med Sci. 1908; 135:342-346.

3. May R, Thurner J. The cause of the predominantly sinistral occurrence of thrombosis of the pelvic veins. Angiology. 1957; 8(5): 419-428.

4. Ehrich WE, Krumbhaar EB. A frequent obstructive anomaly of the mouth of the left common iliac vein. Am Heart J. 1943; 26:737-750.

5. Negus D, Fletcher EW, Cockett FB, Thomas ML. Compression and band formation at the mouth of the left common iliac vein. Br J Surg. 1968; 55: 369-374.

6. Kibbe MR, Ujiki M, Goodwin AL, et al. Iliac vein compression in an asymptomatic patient population. J Vasc Surg. 2004; 39:937-943.

7. Raju S, Neglen P. High prevalence of nonthrombotic iliac vein lesions in chronic venous disease: a permissive role in pathogenicity. J Vasc Surg. 2006; 44: 136- 143.

8. Johnson BF, Manzo RA, Bergelin RD, et al. Relationship between changes in the deep venous system and the development of the postthrombotic syndrome after an acute episode of lower limb deep vein thrombosis: A one- to six-year follow-up. J Vasc Surg. 1995; 21: 307-312.

9. Johnson BF, Manzo RA, Bergelin RD, et al. The site of residual abnormalities in the leg veins in long-term follow-up after deep vein thrombosis and their relationship to the development of the post-thrombotic syndrome. Int Angiol. 1996; 15(1) :14-19.

10. Neglen P, Raju S. Proximal Lower Extremity Chronic Venous Outflow Obstruction: Recognition and Treatment. Semin Vasc Surg.2002; 15(1): 57-64

11. Neglén P, Raju S. Intravascular ultrasound scan evaluation of the obstructed vein. J Vasc Surg. 2002; 35: 694-700.

12. Barwell JR, Davies CE, Deacon F, et al. Comparison of surgery and compression with compression alone in chronic venous ulceration (ESCHAR study): randomised controlled trial. Lancet. 2004; 363(9424):1854-9

13. Oguzkurt L, Tercan F, Pourbagher MA, et al. Computed tomography findings in 10 cases of iliac vein compression (May-Thurner) syndrome. Eur J Radiol. 2005; 55: 421–5

14. Jeon UB, Chung JW, Jae HJ, et al. May-Thurner syndrome complicated by acute iliofemoral vein thrombosis: helical CT venography for evaluation of long-term stent patency and changes in the iliac vein. AJR Am J Roentgenol. 2010; 195: 751-7

15. Fraser DG, Moody AR, Morgan PS, Martel A. Iliac compression syndrome and recanalization of femoropopliteal and iliac venous thrombosis: a prospective study with magnetic resonance venography. J Vasc Surg. 2004; 40(4): 612-9.

16. Wolpert LM, Rahmani O, Stein B, Gallagher JJ, Drezner AD. Magnetic resonance venography in the diagnosis and management of May-Thurner syndrome. Vasc Endovascular Surg. 2002; 36(1): 51-7.

17. Asciutto G, Mumme A, Marpe B, Köster O, Asciutto KC, Geier B. MR venography in the detection of pelvic venous congestion. Eur J Vasc Endovasc Surg. 2008; 36(4): 491-6.

18. Forauer AR, Gemmete JJ, Dasika NL, Cho KJ, Williams DM. Intravascular ultrasound in the diagnosis and treatment of iliac vein compression (May-Thurner) syndrome. J Vasc Interv Radiol. 2002; 13: 523-7.

19. Neglen P, Raju S. Balloon Dilation and Stenting of Chronic Iliac Vein Obstruction: Technical Aspects and Early Clinical Outcome. J Endovasc Ther. 2000; 7(2): 79-91.

20. Juhan C, Hartung O, Alimi Y, Barthélemy P, Valerio N, Portier F. Treatment of nonmalignant obstructive iliocaval lesions by stent placement: mid-term results. Ann Vasc Surg. 2001; 15(2): 227-32.

21. Neglén P, Hollis KC, Olivier J, Raju S. Stenting of the venous outflow in chronic venous disease: long-term stent-related outcome, clinical, and hemodynamic result. J Vasc Surg. 2007;46(5):979-990.

22. Hartung O, Loundou AD, Barthelemy P, Arnoux D, Boufi M, Alimi YS. Endovascular management of chronic disabling ilio-caval obstructive lesions: long-term results. Eur J Vasc Endovasc Surg. 2009; 38: 118-24.

23. Knipp BS, Ferguson E, Williams DM, Dasika NJ, Cwikiel W, Henke PK, et al. Factors associated with outcome after interventional treatment of symptomatic iliac vein compression syndrome. J Vasc Surg. 2007; 46: 743-9.

24. Garg N, Gloviczki P, Karimi KM, Duncan AA, Bjarnason H, Kalra M, et al. Factors affecting outcome of open and hybrid reconstructions for nonmalignant obstruction of iliofemoral veins and inferior vena cava. J Vasc Surg. 2011; 53: 383-93.

25. Alhalbouni S, Hingorani A, Shiferson A, et al. Iliac-femoral venous stenting for lower extremity venous stasis symptoms. Ann Vasc Surg. 2012; 26(2): 185-9.

26. Rosales A, Sandbaek G, Jørgensen JJ. Stenting for chronic post-thrombotic vena cava and iliofemoral venous occlusions: mid-term patency and clinical outcome. Eur J Vasc Endovasc Surg. 2010; 40(2): 234-40.

27. Raju S, Neglen P. Percutaneous recanalization of total occlusions of the iliac vein. J Vasc Surg. 2009; 50: 360-8.

28. Kolbel T, Lindh M, Akesson M, Wasselius J, Gottsater A, Ivancev K. Chronic iliac vein

occlusion: midterm results of endovascular recanalization. J Endovasc Ther. 2009; 16: 483-91.

29. Gutzeit A, Zollikofer ChL, Dettling-Pizzolato M, Graf N, Largiadèr J, Binkert CA. Endovascular stent treatment for symptomatic benign iliofemoral venous occlusive disease: long-term results 1987-2009. Cardiovasc Intervent Radiol. 2011; 34: 542-9.

30. Hartung O, Loundou AD, Barthelemy P, Arnoux D, Boufi M, Alimi YS. Endovascular management of chronic disabling ilio-caval obstructive lesions: long-term results. Eur J Vasc Endovasc Surg. 2009; 38: 118-24.

31. Knipp BS, Ferguson E, Williams DM, Dasika NJ, Cwikiel W, Henke PK, et al. Factors associated with outcome after interventional treatment of symptomatic iliac vein compression syndrome. J Vasc Surg. 2007; 46: 743-9.

32. Meng QY, Li XQ, Qian AM, Sang HF, Rong JJ, Zhu LW. Endovascular treatment of iliac vein compression syndrome. Chin Med J (Engl). 2011; 124: 3281-4.

33. Gloviczki P, Cho JS. Surgical treatment of chronic deep venous obstruction. In: Rutherford RB, ed. Vascular Surgery. 5th edn. New York: Elsevier, 2001: 2099–165

34. Jost CJ, Gloviczki P, Cherry KJ Jr, et al. Surgical reconstruction of iliofemoral veins and the inferior vena cava for nonmalignant occlusive disease. J Vasc Surg. 2001;33(2): 320–7.

35. Gloviczki P, Kalra M, Duncan AA, Oderich GS, Vrtiska TJ, Bower TC. Open and hybrid deep vein reconstructions: to do or not to do? Phlebology. 2012; 27 Suppl 1:103-6.

36. Alimi Y, Hartung O.Iliocaval Venous Obstruction: Surgical Treatment in Cronenwett J, Johnston KW ed. Rutherford's Vascular Surgery 7th edn. Philadelphia: Elsevier, 2010: 919-945

37. Robison RJ, Peigh PS, Fiore AC, et al: Venous prostheses: improved patency with external stents. J Surg Res. 1984; 36 (4) :306-311.

38. Dalsing MC, Raju S, Wakefield TW, Taheri S: A multicenter, phase I evaluation of cryopreserved venous valve allografts for the treatment of chronic deep venous insufficiency. J Vasc Surg. 1999; 30:854-864.

39. Gloviczki P, Pairolero PC: Venous reconstruction for obstruction and valvular incompetence. Perspect Vasc Surg. 1988; 1:75-93.

40. Alimi YS, DiMauro P, Fabre D, Juhan C: Iliac vein reconstructions to treat acute and chronic venous occlusive disease. J Vasc Surg. 1997; 25:673-681.

41. Dale WA, Harris J, Terry RB: Polytetrafluoroethylene reconstruction of the inferior vena cava. Surgery. 1984; 95:625-630.

42. Kunlin K, Kunlin A: Experimental venous surgery. In: May R, ed. Surgery of the Veins of the Leg and Pelvis, Philadelphia, PA: WB Saunders; 1979:37-75.

43. Yamaguchi A, Eguchi S, Iwasaki T, Asano K: The influence of arteriovenous fistulae on the patency of synthetic inferior vena caval grafts. J Cardiovasc Surg. 1968; 9:99-103.

44. Gloviczki P, Hollier LH, Dewanjee MK, et al: Experimental replacement of the inferior vena cava: factors affecting patency. Surgery. 1984; 95:657-666.

45.   Menawat SS, Gloviczki P, Mozes G, et al: Effect of a femoral arteriovenous fistula on lower extremity venous hemodynamics after femorocaval reconstruction. J Vasc Surg. 1996; 24:793-799.

46.   Palma EC, Riss F, Del Campo F, Tobler H: Tratamiento de los trastornos postflebiticos mediante anastomosis venosa safeno-femoral cotrolateral. Bull Soc Surg Uruguay. 1958; 29:135-145.

47.   Palma EC, Esperon R: Vein transplants and grafts in the surgical treatment of the postphlebitic syndrome. J Cardiovasc Surg. 1960; 1:94-107.

48.   Halliday P, Harris J, May J: Femoro-femoral crossover grafts (Palma operation): a long-term follow-up study. In: Bergan JJ, Yao JST, ed. Surgery of the Veins, Orlando, FL: Grune & Stratton; 1985:241-254.

49.   AbuRahma AF, Robinson PA, Boland JP: Clinical hemodynamic and anatomic predictors of long-term outcome of lower extremity venovenous bypasses. J Vasc Surg. 1991; 14:635-644.

Chapter 19

Popliteal Vein Compression Syndrome: Diagnosis and Management

Author(s)
Dr Richard Harris
Mr Michael Cuzzilla

Institution(s)
Kuring-Gai Vascular Specialists, Sydney Adventist Hospital and Hornsby Hospital, Suite G05, 10 Edgeworth David Avenue, Hornsby NSW Australia 2077

Introduction

Syndromes are fascinating. A collection of signs and symptoms that pull together to create an entity. Hopefully, one that can be successfully managed. Sometimes, it is not until a syndrome is pointed out by an expert that you can see it. Sometimes, collections of symptoms sit quietly in a physician's mind and are not collated, just noted. When the group of criteria that define a syndrome are laid out, suddenly you recognise it clearly all of the time. Such is my experience with popliteal vein compression syndrome (PVCS). It has become one of those entities that I now see very clearly in my practice but which I had previously understood and managed poorly. In the literature, there is information regarding this syndrome including detailed espousals of anatomical variants and confusing parallels with popliteal artery entrapment syndromes. However, there is little or no literature yet on the very modern and simple ways of recognising this syndrome and the simple way it can now be managed.

If you have a significant vein practice and you understand the pathophysiology you will see these patients every week in your clinic. You will check for this syndrome with every single ultrasound study and you will treat these patients regularly with appropriate surgical decompression before you consider ablating any additional superficial venous reflux.

Extrinsic compression of the popliteal vein, but not the associated clinical syndrome, was described by Nicolaides et al. in 1992[1]. This study outlined the functional obstruction that occurs in a significant number of otherwise healthy patients without previous history of DVT.

This clearly begs the questions: "What is the PVCS?", "How was it discovered?" and "How is it best treated?"

What exactly is the popliteal vein compression syndrome (PVCS)?

PVCS is a clinical finding of lower limb venous hypertension due to partial or complete obstruction of the popliteal vein in the upright patient, with the knee in the straight locked position. This phenomenon is increasingly found in obese populations. Complete obstruction of the popliteal vein in this position is found in 5% of a typical western population with partial obstruction seen in a further 10%.

The mechanism of action is compression of the vein usually over a 2-4 cm segment via tension produced by the popliteal fascia in the twisting motion of knee locking, relaxation of the gastrocnemius muscle and hence increased bulk and a high fat content of the popliteal fossa in this usually obese patient cohort (Figure 1).

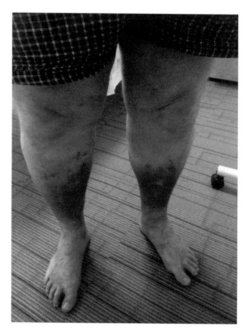

Figure 1: Typical patient presenting with PVCS. Note the significant circumferential hyperpigmentation and obviously high BMI.

The patient that walks into your clinic or surgery with this condition is usually, but not universally, significantly overweight. Symptoms are induced by standing and the clinical and ultrasound examination will often be negative for reflux and will be negative for intrinsic fixed obstruction. The patient complains often of leg swelling, heaviness and tiredness. Almost all patients with a clinically significant PVCS will avoid having their legs in the straight position. For example they will avoid standing still for long periods of time and when sitting, will bend their knees to avoid symptoms. This also applies when they are in bed where again they will avoid having their legs in the straight position. Often these patients present with significant signs and symptoms including pain and aching, severe circumferential pigmentation, submalleolar flaring, fat necrosis, atrophie blanche and ulceration. Inflammation in the gaiter region is very typical.

Of great concern to the Vascular Specialist who is dealing with veins regularly will be the patient who has previously presented elsewhere and had stripping or ablation of their great and/or small saphenous veins in the context of what you recognise as PVCS. Alarm bells will be ringing for often these patients complain that their symptoms have significantly worsened since that ablative procedure. It is imperative to recognise and treat PVCS before embarking on superficial reflux procedures. The problem arises almost certainly because a superficial route of escape for the high venous pressures generated distally by extrinsic compression of the popliteal vein is removed by ablation. Patients may attend with markedly worse signs of venous hypertension, possibly ulceration and worsening of the original symptoms.

Another feature seen when the superficial reflux is dealt with prior to PVCS being addressed is early superficial venous recurrence. This is seen particularly in the lower leg and usually takes the form of development of multiple incompetent perforator veins. An aggressive perforator incompetence may be encountered.

Early understanding and history of recognition and treatment

A single patient with this syndrome sparked interest by a specialist Vascular Sonographer who reported the findings to the Vascular Surgeon in the practice. The patient was an obese female who had marked clinical signs of venous hypertension without any apparent venous reflux. Whilst it was not in the protocol at the time, the sonographer, Michael Cuzzilla, noted that the patient was occluding their popliteal vein when their leg was in the locked straight position (Figure 2). In the absence of any other explanation for the venous hypertensive changes the sonographer, with many years of exposure to a large venous cohort, managed to put two and two together.

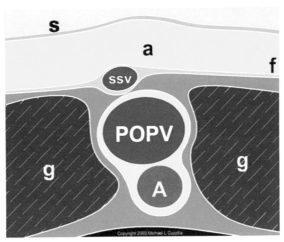

Figure 2A: Mechanism of obstruction of popliteal vein. Cross-sectional schematics of popliteal fossa-Baseline. Key: s=skin, a = adipose tissue; ssv = small saphenous vein; f =fascia; POPV = popliteal vein, A = popliteal artery, g = gastrocnemius muscle

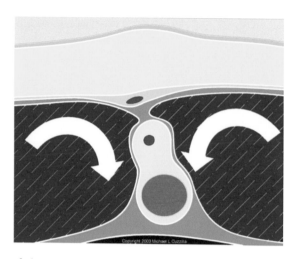

Figure 2B: Mechanism of obstruction of popliteal vein. Cross-sectional schematics of popliteal fossa-Knee Locked

It was then left to the Vascular Surgeon, Professor Rodney Lane to develop a strategy to deal with this presentation. Arterial and venous compression had been described before. These descriptions mainly reported anatomical variations and had prompted surgical solutions that were quite invasive.

Lane et al.[1] reported success using a large sigmoid incision in the popliteal fossa with complete dissection of the popliteal vein and leaving the fascial wound open. Closure at the skin level was performed. This study first linked an abnormally large BMI to the presence of the PVCS, demonstrating an average BMI of 34.6 compared to 25.3 in a group of normal venous reflux patients. It also demonstrated that surgical decompression improved popliteal vein diameter when the knee was in the locked position, from an average of 1 mm^2 to 9 mm^2. A further link between increased body mass index and PVCS was established by Huber[2].

This extensive surgical decompression, whilst successful, resulted in a very painful recovery. It was usual to have a stay in hospital of at least two nights and it was not infrequent to have post-operative problems of haematoma, wound infection or a lymphatic leak as a consequence of the procedure. The patient usually required two weeks off work. However 99% of patients were reported to have had successful popliteal decompression, making it possible to deal with the superficial venous disease either at the same time or shortly thereafter.

In the context of a move to more minimally invasive surgery for venous disease and the onset of the endovenous ablative techniques coming into use, I explored a new approach to popliteal decompression in 2009. The technique will be described in the final section.

Diagnosis

It is my belief that every single ultrasound study for the investigation of lower limb venous disease should include an assessment for PVCS. This should include greyscale measurements of the cross-sectional area (mm^2) of the popliteal vein with the patient in the standing position (Figure 3). Two measurements are required, one with the knee slightly flexed and the second when the knee is locked straight as when standing. If there is no diminution of the popliteal vein diameter on real-time greyscale imaging, which will be the case in the vast majority of patients, then a simple note that no abnormality was detected can be recorded on the venous ultrasound worksheet and subsequent report. However, if there is a decrease in the area of the vessel, which is initially assessed in the longitudinal plane and then more specifically addressed in a transverse plane, then the cross-sectional area should be recorded in both positions in both legs.

If one leg is being assessed and partial or complete PVCS is being demonstrated, then it is very sensible to go on to assess the contralateral leg for a similar abnormality.

This abnormality should not be looked for in isolation. Full insonation and assessment of the function of the deep veins and the superficial venous systems should be performed as standard. Popliteal Vein Compression Syndrome is certainly associated with a higher risk for DVT and so post-phlebitic changes may be demonstrated but is not pathognomonic. There is also a higher risk for perforator vein incompetence distal to the popliteal vein. In association with superficial reflux the clinical signs associated with venous hypertension may be accelerated.

There is a significant group of patients where popliteal vein compression is demonstrated on ultrasound but who have no significant superficial venous disease and little evidence of venous hypertensive changes. There is absolutely no indication for intervention in these patients unless they are significantly symptomatic in other respects. Many patients will be simply able to be educated about the condition and asked to return if any signs or symptoms of venous hypertension become apparent.

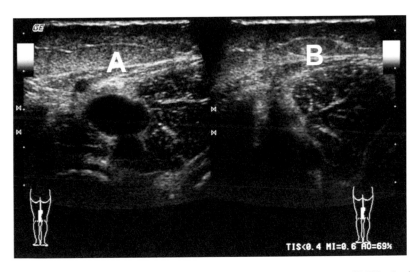

Figure 3: Grey scale ultrasound imaging of the popliteal vein demonstrating positive PVCS. In the baseline image (A) the popliteal vein is widely patent as opposed to during locking of the knee when the popliteal vein lumen is completely occluded (B).

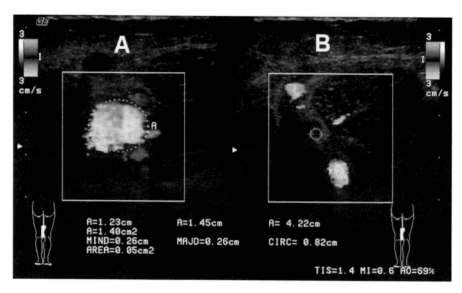

Figure 4: A Colour Doppler image demonstrating the presence of PVCS as indicated by variations to the baseline lumen (A), where both a decrease in the cross-sectional area measurement and the absence of colour flow in the popliteal vein during knee locking (B) can be observed.

Of course greyscale ultrasound is used to interrogate other anatomical variants such as popliteal vein duplication, small saphenous termination and function, exclusion or documentation of thrombophlebitic changes, musculo-skeletal abnormalities which may contribute to symptoms such as Baker's cysts and popliteal artery aneurysm disease. In looking for the PVCS a longitudinal sweep of the popliteal fossae is made from the adductor hiatus to the upper calf with the calf slightly flexed. The maximal cross-sectional area of the vein at the popliteal crease is documented by recording diameters in the transverse plane using callipers and standard ultrasound software. The patient is then told to adopt a position of comfortable extension with the knee locked straight. A similar sweep of the popliteal vein segment is undertaken and diameters and luminal area recorded. Abnormal obstructive flow spectral waveform patterns in the distal popliteal vein and/or calf vessels will be noted if there is a complete popliteal vein compression in this position (Figure 4).

Treatment

The patient with a complete or near complete PVCS (area in straight leg position less than 2 mm^2) and either superficial reflux that will need to be dealt with or significant symptoms directly related to their PVCS will need to be considered for operative management.

The original operation performed was based on procedures similar to those required for dealing with popliteal arterial entrapment syndromes and originally performed by Professor Rod Lane. This involved a large sigmoid incision with the upper component lateral, a transverse component based on the popliteal crease and a medial component inferiorly.

This original procedure involved incision of the popliteal fascia, sometimes minimal removal of popliteal fossae fat, careful dissection of the entire affected area of popliteal vein to the adventitia with particular care for nerve preservation and occasionally division of the medial head of gastrocnemius. A suction drain was placed near the vessels and the wound was sutured closed just at the skin level, leaving the fascial division open. It was a relatively painful operation from which to recover and as stated above, the patients generally stayed two nights post-operatively, had a painful recovery and risks of haematoma, wound infection or lymphatic leak.

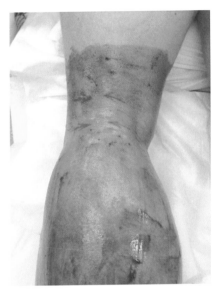

Figure 5: Preparation of the patient in the prone position. Note the ultrasound guided markings (arrows) performed the day prior to procedure to identify the anatomic site of maximal compression.

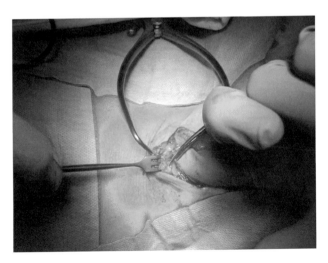

Figure 6: Careful division of the popliteal fossa with finger protection of underlying structures along the entire length of the incision.

In March 2009 in a venous world becoming oriented to minimally invasive approaches and in particular coinciding with my handling an increasing number of patients with superficial venous reflux with outpatient endovenous laser ablation rather than an open surgical approach, I decided to trial a new operative procedure for PVCS. The key to this approach was to pre-operatively identify and very accurately mark the site of maximal popliteal vein compression with ultrasound (Figure 5). This is usually done the day before the surgery. Vein markings for small saphenous ligation and stripping may be considered but great saphenous reflux is usually left for a later session of outpatient endovenous laser ablation.

With this new procedure a small transverse incision is made at the site of the marked maximal popliteal vein compression. This is usually around 3 cm in length. Incision is made thorough the superficial fat and a transverse incision carefully made through the popliteal fascia. Very careful and precise lifting of the fascia is then undertaken with a finger placed directly under the fascia (Figure 6) with a Metzenbaum scissor used to split the fascia vertically both proximally and distally. The fasciotomy is carried out to beyond a point of restriction felt in the popliteal fascia. This is hard to define in text but quite obvious intra-operatively. Usually the fasciotomy is 6 or 7 cm in length in both directions. Care is undertaken to achieve excellent haemostasis and to ensure that all fascial layers and bands have been divided. Finger protection of the underlying structures is essential throughout the fasciotomy. The wound is closed using subcuticular sutures and Steristrips™ only at the skin layer. A Primapore™ dressing is applied and overnight the patient is placed into a toe to above knee compression bandage.

Post-operatively the patient's level of discomfort in comparison to the original procedure is greatly diminished with most people not even requiring paracetamol by the next day. A below-knee compression stocking is utilised continuously for 7 days and for another week following that during the day. Outpatient ablative procedures are usually performed around 5 or 6 weeks post operatively if required.

A standard ultrasound study confirming elimination of the PVCS routine is mandatory prior to any ablative procedure. Other authors emphasise venographic studies in the context of chronic venous insufficiency investigations where other causes have been excluded. The older style procedure was recommended and as expected decompression was achieved in all patients[3].

The success of this procedure technically in terms of eliminating the PVCS is very similar to the original larger procedure. However recovery and return to work is dramatically faster with this approach. Complications like wound haematoma or lymph leak are virtually eliminated.

In 78 patients treated with the new procedure the PVCS was eliminated in all patients of which 76 had both symptomatic and technical relief. One required the older procedure to achieve this and one had symptomatic and functional relief but on ultrasound had persisting compression of the popliteal vein. There were no nerve or wound complications of the procedure.

References

1.   Leon M, Volteas N Nicolaides AN. Popliteal vein entrapment in the normal population. Eur

J Vasc Surg. 1992; 6 (6):623-7

2. Huber DE, Huber JP. Popliteal vein compression under general anaesthesia. Eur J Vasc Endovasc Surg. 2009; 37 (4):464-9.

3. R J Lane, M L Cuzzilla, R A Harris, M N Phillips. Popliteal vein compression syndrome: obesity, venous disease and the popliteal connection. Phlebology. 2009; 24(5): 201-207.

4. Raju S, Neglen P. Popliteal vein entrapment: A benign venographic feature or a pathologic entity. J Vasc Surg. 2000; 31:631-41.

Chapter 20

Assessing the IVC and Iliac Veins with IVUS and Indications for Deep Venous Stenting

Author
Seshadri Raju

Institution
The Rane Center for Lymphatic and Venous Diseases, Jackson. MS. USA

Introduction

The iliac-caval veins are central to lower limb outflow and are hemodynamically important in chronic venous disease. Post-thrombotic involvement of iliac veins had been known for more than two centuries. The father of modern pathology, Carl Von Rokitanski (1804-1878) described in detail the pathologic changes that occur in these vessels from autopsy studies. McMurrich, a Canadian pathologist, described in 1905 a different kind of lesion – a spur or web – that occurred at the iliac-caval junction underneath the right iliac artery where it crossed it. That lesion is now known to be of non-thrombotic origin and is likely caused by the repetitive trauma of the closely-related pulsating artery. In some instances, the lesions may be ontogenic. A number of eponymous titles (May-Thurner Syndrome; Cockett Syndrome) are attached to the syndrome, so designated for those who raised awareness of the lesion. It is also commonly referred to as 'iliac compression syndrome', a misnomer in that compression is but a part of the complex lesion which also involves intraluminal webs and wall fibrosis. "Non-thrombotic iliac vein lesion (NIVL)" is probably a better nomenclature[1].

Cockett[2] popularized the notion that the syndrome primarily affected the left lower extremity of young women with manifestation of swelling and pain, often exacerbated by onset of secondary thrombosis[3] at the obstructive site. From use of modern diagnostic techniques, we now know that in fact NIVL affects both sexes, both lower limbs and the median age is in fact older in the fifties. The condition has excited interest and sometimes intense controversy, not surprising because of the many unique features associated with it. To begin with, the lesion occurs in silent form (ie. asymptomatic) in a significant percentage of the normal population. Early autopsy findings[4] and more recent imaging studies[5] have established that the lesion occurs in as many as 60% of the general population. Many have argued that a lesion so ubiquitous and so commonly silent cannot possibly be pathological. In fact some radiology texts describe the lesion and the collaterals associated with it as a 'normal anatomical variant'. It is, however, difficult to determine how the body knows to recognize a severe central venous stenosis with collaterals as a 'normal' variant!

A more rational explanation is to view the obstructive lesion as 'permissive' – silent at the moment with potential to decompensate into the symptomatic version with additional insults to the limb, such as trauma, cellulitis, thrombosis (DVT), or onset of reflux with age (Table 1). In many symptomatic patients, history of a precipitating insult such as recent knee surgery can be elicited. Post-thrombotic iliac vein lesions sustained from a prior episode of deep venous thrombosis can remain dormant until a second episode of thrombosis or other insult to precipitates symptoms (Figure 1).

- Trauma
- Infection
- Reflux (incidence^ age)
- DVT
- Joint surgery
- Seated orthostasis and poor calf pump (elderly)
- Obesity
- Edematogenic meds.
- Postmenopausal hormonal changes
- Lymphatic damage from vein disease itself or from, cancer, radiation, chemo, surgery.

Table 1: Secondary insults that may precipitate symptoms in the presence of a silent iliac vein lesion.

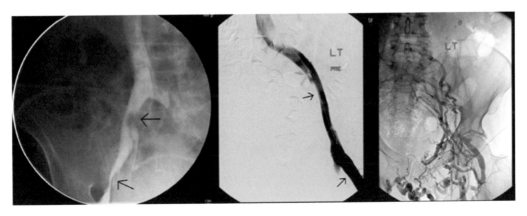

Figure 1: Post-thrombotic lesions sustained years or even decades ago can become symptomatic if there is a precipitating cause listed in Table 1. Post-thrombotic lesions shown above had been present for several years before symptoms developed. Arrows point to focal stenosis (left) and diffuse iliac stenosis (middle) with a caliber smaller than the femoral vein. The figure on the right shows chronic total occlusion that had remained asymptomatic for several years.

Human pathology is replete with such permissive lesions. A classic example is the foramen ovale with a silent incidence of ≈25% in the general population. A tiny fraction will eventually become symptomatic with onset of paradoxical embolus. Other permissive/pathologic combinations include obesity/diabetes, hypertension/stroke; carotid plaque/transient ischemic attacks, ureteral reflux/ pyelonephritis, Helicobacter/peptic ulcer and many others. In each case, the permissive lesion occurs in silent form in a certain percentage of the general population, progressing to overt disease in a smaller subset. The incidence of the permissive lesion in the symptomatic subset is much higher than the silent incidence.

A general principle of treatment of these lesions is to treat or eliminate the permissive lesion first, which often proves curative. Specific attention to secondary pathology will be required only when the general approach fails. For example, weight reduction is the first choice of treatment in secondary diabetes and the elimination of Helicobacter in peptic ulcer. Correction of NIVL will often relieve symptoms including healing of the stasis ulceration, even if the associated reflux remains uncorrected[6].

Correction of iliac vein obstructive lesions has become simpler with introduction of minimally invasive stent technology, which requires only outpatient admission. Treated patients recover quickly, the morbidity is minor and stent patency is astonishingly high (much higher than in iliac arteries) with commensurate symptom relief. These obvious advantages have rendered open surgery often extensive and complex with much higher morbidity and failure rate, obsolete. In major centers in the USA open surgery is now performed only as a salvage maneuver after the stent procedure has failed.

Patient Selection for Iliac Vein Stenting

Chronic venous disease (CVD) is a multisystem disease of varying severity involving one or more of the superficial, deep and perforator venous systems. With advancing severity of the disease reflected by the CEAP clinical class, more systems, each of increasing severity, tend to be involved[7,8]. A curious and unique feature of CVD is that partial correction of multivarious pathology can remit the disease even when uncorrected pathology remains. Minimally invasive techniques of correcting each of these system pathologies are now available. This means a new treatment paradigm is available wherein simpler techniques can be employed first before progressing to more complex treatment options until disease remission is achieved. Certain clinical patterns and quantitative analysis of system pathology can predict correction of which of the three systems is likely to yield the greatest benefit, providing a guideline of sequential order of interventions. In some instances, where there is uncertainty as to the severity of one or the other systems in pathogenesis, combined treatments can be provided in a single setting because the techniques are minimally invasive.

The higher efficacy and safety profile of venous stenting allow a broader spectrum of patients to be considered for venous stenting than would be the case for open surgical procedures. Even octogenarians tolerate the procedure well without mortality[9]. Generally, patients with CEAP clinical class 3 and higher are candidates. This means patients with leg swelling, skin manifestations such as dermatitis or venous ulcers who have failed compression therapy will be considered (Figure 2).

A subclass that can benefit are those patients with recurrent cellulitis of the limb. Swelling may be mild or even absent initially but increases in severity with repetitive attacks of cellulitis. Recurrent cellulitis is damaging to lymphatics. Chronic venous disease in general (even without cellulitis) leads to damage to the pre-collector or small lymphatics[10]. The mechanism is unknown but approximately 30% of patients with chronic venous disease will show abnormal lymphoscintographic findings[11]. It is not uncommon for such patients to assume clinical features such as squaring of toes, swelling of the dorsum of the foot, non-pinch ability of the toe skin (Stemmer sign), which are said to be characteristic of lymphedema. Venous lymphedema arising from venous obstruction is probably more common than the 'primary' lymphedema variety, simply because of the high prevalence of venous pathology in the general population. It is likely many such patients with potentially correctible venous lesions go without treatment, because they are not adequately investigated and the diagnosis is missed.

Venous limb pain is among the most common and most disabling features of venous disease[12]. Current CEAP classification does not adequately represent the spectrum of venous symptoms that fall under the pain category. These include heaviness of the limb when the limb is dependent (sitting or standing), restless legs, leg cramps and diffuse limb pain of varying severity. Elevation of the limb and calf pump action ("walking off the pain") ameliorate or relieve the pain symptoms. In some patients venous pain manifestations are atypical and distinguishing the venous origin from arterial or other causes of pain may be difficult even after investigations. In some patients, leg pain, restless legs or cramps occur mostly at night after they have "gotten off their feet" decoupling the pathognomonic association of pain with leg dependency in CVD.

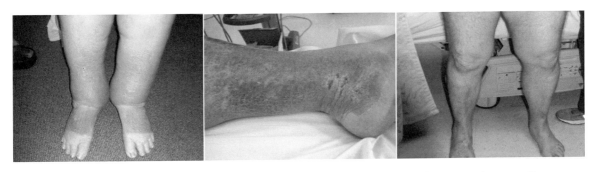

Figure 2: Clinical indications for venous stenting. Leg swelling (left) and stasis ulceration with surrounding dermatitis (middle). Patient with venous hypertension syndrome (right); note absence of clinical signs of venous disease with normal appearance of the leg (see text).

Venous claudication which exacerbates pain with walking or climbing stairs is associated with severe obstruction or chronic total occlusions (CTO) and may require arterial as well as venous investigations to identify the correct etiology. Most difficult are patients whose only symptom manifestation is orthostatic venous pain with no other venous history (prior DVT, for example) or distinguishing venous clinical signs such as varicosities or skin changes that might point the diagnosis toward the venous system (Figure 2). A careful history that identifies the pain with the erect posture is often the only clue as to the correct diagnosis of "venous hypertension syndrome." Pain disproportionate to signs should include CVD in the differential diagnosis. It is not unusual for this type of patient with 'venous hypertension syndrome' to make the rounds of many physicians' offices without a correct diagnosis and perhaps even be mislabeled as suffering from psychosomatic pain!

Treatment Algorithm

Since CVD seldom poses a threat to life or limb most patients will initially be treated conservatively with compression and ancillary measures before interventional procedures are considered. This does not mean, however, that patients are subjected to compression for years on end before providing interventional relief. A trial of compression for perhaps 2 to 3 months should be enough to gauge its efficacy[13]. Dominant deep venous pathology frequently does not yield to conservative relief.

It is useful to perform a thorough duplex examination at the outset to define the underlying pathology and provide an estimation of whether conservative treatment will be successful. The clinical presentation combined with a detailed duplex examination can provide the framework of a suitable treatment plan[12] for the individual patient, taking into account the CVD pathology and relevant socioeconomic factors. Younger patients will require return to work sooner and older patients may not be able to use certain treatment options. For instance, frailty or arthritis may preclude effective compression over extended duration without institutionalization. Specific pathologic correction can obviate the need for permanent compression[13]. If the chief complaint is varices with local symptoms, the clinical attention need not go beyond the superficial venous system (mini phlebectomy/saphenous ablation) regardless of whether there is pathology in the deep system. If the pain is diffuse involving the limb or there are systemic symptoms such as leg cramps or restless legs, significant saphenous reflux and deep venous pathology (obstruction/reflux) are usually present. The size of the refluxive saphenous vein can indicate if its refluxive component is significant. Clinical experience and Poisueille law (flow related to 4th power of radius) suggest that a saphenous vein <5 mm in size is unlikely to harbor serious reflux (volume). In that case, deep venous reflux is the main culprit.

If no deep venous reflux is detectable on duplex, iliac vein obstruction is likely present. Current duplex methodology is poorly sensitive to this obstructive pathology. Venography (about 50% sensitive)[4,14] can be helpful if positive, but intravascular ultrasound examination (IVUS) may be needed to detect and aid in correction of iliac vein stenosis. Combined saphenous ablation and iliac vein stenting[15] is the procedure of choice if reflux is present in a small (e.g. 3 mm) saphenous vein combined with iliac vein obstruction. Both procedures can be carried out safely in the same session.

Advanced CVD symptoms such as leg swelling beyond ankledema, lipodermatosis, stasis dermatitis or frank ulceration are seldom caused by saphenous reflux alone (except rarely when the saphenous size is ≥10 mm) and deep system involvement is almost always present. If initial 'trial' ablation of a large saphena is elected initially in such cases because of its relative simplicity, the patient may be warned in advance that deep system intervention may be required if the initial approach fails to yield clinical relief.

Combined obstruction (iliac) and reflux (infrainguinal) is the most common deep system pathology to be encountered. Pure obstruction without reflux is found in about a third of patients[1,6]. This can be of post thrombotic or non-thrombotic etiology.

Correction of reflux has dominated therapeutic algorithms in the past century. Attention to correction of obstruction is attracting increasing scrutiny because it can be corrected minimally-invasively with recently introduced stent technology. Even chronic total occlusions of the iliac-caval-femoral vein segments (CTO) can be recanalized[16,17]. This daunting pathology previously required complex open surgery. Valve repair requires rather intricate open technique and is available only in select centers.

Initial experience with venous stenting for obstruction has yielded some surprising clinical observations. In combined obstruction/reflux, initial stent correction of the obstructive component yields such excellent symptom relief to an extent that correction of reflux is not required afterwards— the residual reflux is well tolerated without symptoms in the majority of patients[1,6,13]. This highlights the importance of obstructive pathology vis à vis reflux underlying CVD symptomatology[18,19]. Stent failure occurs mostly in CTO recanalizations[9]. Leg ulcers can be recalcitrant even after iliac vein stenting in post-thrombotic patients with extensive reflux involving multiple valve segments[13]. This subset of patients has few easy choices for permanent cure. They are candidates for ablation of perforators underlying the ulcer with sclerotherapy or thermal ablation as pioneered by Whiteley[20,21]. The procedure can be safely repeated in case of initial failure or recurrence.

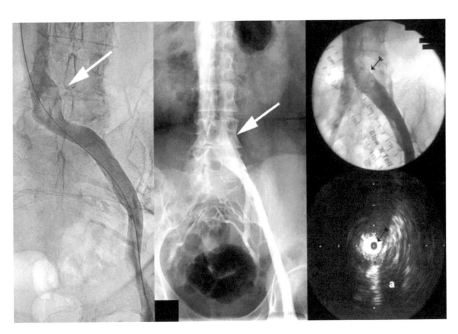

Figure 3: Variable venographic appearance of non-thrombotic iliac vein lesions. Island like translucency in the iliac vein (left) and pancaking of the terminal iliac vein with collaterals (middle). On the right is shown an example where the venogram appears normal but IVUS showed a tight lesion (bottom right). See text.

IVUS Examination

The introduction of intravascular ultrasound (IVUS) has dramatically improved diagnostic accuracy of iliac vein obstruction[22,23]. It is an invaluable tool in placement of the stent as well. Prior venous diagnostics had largely depended on venography, which has poor diagnostic sensitivity in this area. Only about 50% of the lesions can be inferred often by indirect or subtle signs (Figure 3)[1,4,14]. An overt stenosis or obstructive web is only visualized rarely through the flood of contrast. The venogram may appear 'normal' in as many as 30% of cases. Pathologic detail such as perivenous fibrosis, trabeculae, webs and membranes are clearly visible on IVUS (Figure 4) whereas they are more frequently obscured on venography than not. A diffuse form of post thrombotic stenosis, first identified by Rokitanski, can present a 'normal' appearance on venography (Figure 5). This type of lesion occurs in about a third of post-thrombotic cases. Diagnostic IVUS is conveniently combined with stent placement in a single sitting with prior patient consent.

Technique of Iliac Vein Stenting

Details of technique can be found in prior publications[17,24,25]. The technique distinctly differs from arterial applications. For instance, arterial stenting is focused on restoring flow through the lesion. While restoring patency is certainly important, venous stenting should relieve venous hypertension, which is the source of symptoms. This means employing large caliber stents approximating normal anatomy. Use of small caliber stents as in peripheral arterial applications can result in residual symptoms or worse (stent thrombosis) in the CVD patient. This type of complication from undersized stents is often an irretrievable technical error that is not easily corrected.

IVUS is invaluable during stent placement to guide the choice of proper end points for the stent stack. In this respect it is far superior to venography and reduces radiation exposure as well. In the low flow venous system, residual uncorrected lesions retard flow and result in residual symptoms. Unlike in arteries, where minor imperfections are well tolerated due to high velocity flow, all venous lesions both major and minor must be corrected with the stent to achieve optimum flow and distal

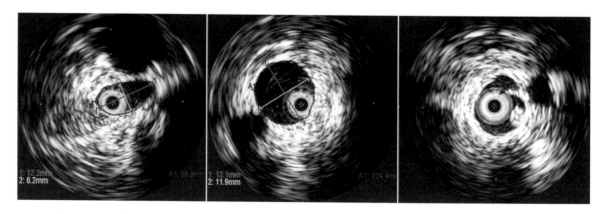

Figure 4: A web as seen on IVUS before and after stenting (left & middle). Trabeculated post-thrombotic vein seen on IVUS (right). Note perivenous fibrosis which will not be visible on venography.

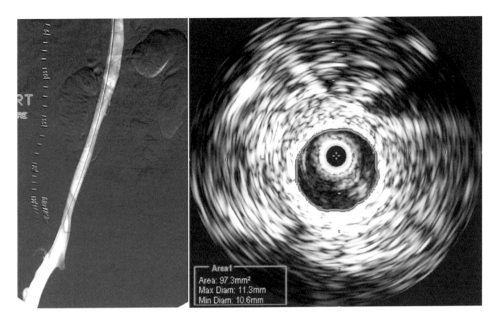

Figure 5: Diffuse iliac vein stenosis can present a normal venographic appearance (left). IVUS shows perivenous fibrosis with luminal stenosis (right). Area measurements can be made with IVUS equipment to accurately assess the extent of stenosis.

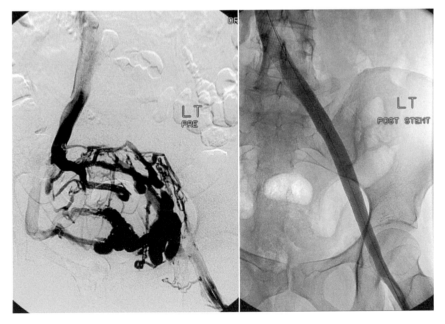

Figure 6: An example of successful recanalization of an iliac vein CTO lesion. Notice the disappearance of collaterals after stenting.

decompression. It is an intuitive belief of many interventionalists that excess of metal (prosthetic length) predisposes to thrombosis. However, counter intuitively, the extent of stenting is less of a concern than uncorrected residual lesions in thrombotic potential. Stent thrombosis is a rare event if the stent stack is free of technical defects and is assured of good inflow and outflow. Stent thrombosis in post-thrombotic limbs (particularly in CTO recanalizations) are more often related to compromised inflow into the stent than inherent thrombophilic potential that may be present in this subset[26]. An example of successful recanalization is shown in Figure 6.

Intraprocedure heparin or Bivalrudin is used but postoperative continuation can be more selective according to the underlying pathology. Most non-thrombotic lesions can be managed with only aspirin for long-term maintenance[9]. In post-thrombotic limbs, long-term anticoagulation for a variable period based on underlying factors that provoked the initial thrombosis can be applied based on current guidelines.

Results

Patency rates (cumulative) in the major subsets undergoing iliac-caval venous stenting are shown in Figure 7. All stent thrombosis occurred only in post-thrombotic limbs, particularly after CTO recanalizations. The rarity of stent thrombosis in the non-thrombotic subset followed long term is an astonishing statistic. Even in post-thrombotic limbs with thrombogenic potential, patency is generally higher than in arterial experience. Counter to expectations, the venous environment is not hostile to prosthetic devices despite a low pressure, low velocity flow profile.

Mortality after iliac vein stenting is negligible and the morbidity is minor – mostly transient back pain in about a quarter of the patients, which subsides in a few days with outpatient analgesics. Complications are few. The incidence of post-stent deep vein thrombosis ($\approx$3% $\leq$30 days) is in line with other vascular interventions. Late (>30 days) deep venous thrombosis mirrors interval thrombotic incidence ($\approx$7%) expected in the post-thrombotic population. About 20% of stented patients may require subsequent re-interventions to correct in-stent restenosis, which has a lower incidence ($\approx$5%) than in arterial stenting[27,28]. The high patency rates are reflected in corresponding symptom relief (Figure 8). QOL parameters improve significantly (data not shown). Of note, ulcers heal in $\approx$75% (cumulative) with very few recurrences long-term (flat curve) after venous stenting alone even though significant residual reflux remains uncorrected (Figure 9). This is the case even in limbs with reflux variety (axial reflux) that is considered serious in its clinical impact.

Conclusion

IVUS-guided iliac vein stenting is emerging as an attractive minimally invasive therapeutic option with excellent safety and efficacy in a wide spectrum of symptomatic patients with CVD who have failed conservative therapy.

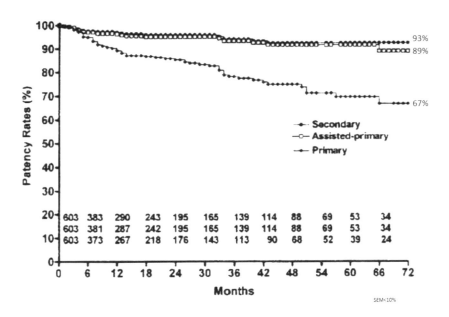

Figure 7: Long term cumulative stent patency. Primary, primary assisted and secondary patencies are separately shown. The curves includes both post-thrombotic and non-thrombotic limbs. Thrombosis in the latter subset is extremely rare (see text). Stent thrombosis is nearly exclusive to post-thrombotic limbs particularly in CTO recanalizations.

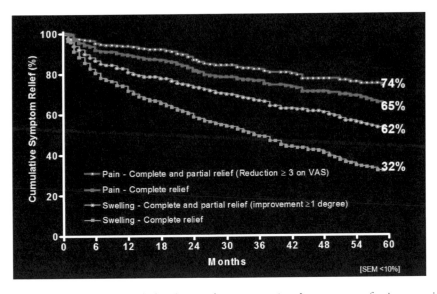

Figure 8: Cumulative symptom relief after iliac-caval venous stenting. Improvement of pain occurs in 74% with complete relief in 65% at 5 years. Corresponding figures for swelling are somewhat less though quite satisfactory.

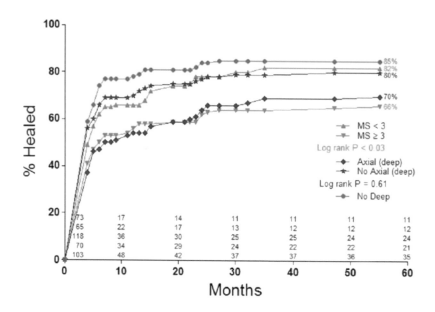

Figure 9: Ulcer healing after iliac vein stent. Cumulative long term curves are shown for subsets without associated reflux, axial reflux and multisegment reflux. The reflux component was not corrected after stent placement. There is no difference between no reflux and axial reflux even though the latter is considered a severe form of reflux. Ulcer healing in subset with reflux in 3 or more valve stations was significantly less but 66% of ulcers healed long term even in this disadvantaged group. If reflux was present in <3 segments, healing was similar to the subset without reflux. Note all curves are flat after initial healing, meaning sparse recurrences.

References

1.   Raju S, Neglen P. High prevalence of nonthrombotic iliac vein lesions in chronic venous disease: a permissive role in pathogenicity. Journal of vascular surgery : official publication, the Society for Vascular Surgery [and] International Society for Cardiovascular Surgery, North American Chapter.2006; 44: 136-43; discussion 44.

2.   Cockett FB, Thomas ML. The iliac compression syndrome. Br J Surg. 1965; 52: 816-21.

3.   Cockett FB, Thomas ML, Negus D. Iliac vein compression.--Its relation to iliofemoral thrombosis and the post-thrombotic syndrome. Br Med J.1967; 2: 14-9.

4.   Negus D, Fletcher EW, Cockett FB, Thomas ML. Compression and band formation at the mouth of the left common iliac vein. Br J Surg. 1968; 55: 369-74.

5.   Kibbe MR, Ujiki M, Goodwin AL, Eskandari M, Yao J, Matsumura J. Iliac vein compression in an asymptomatic patient population. Journal of vascular surgery : official publication, the Society for Vascular Surgery [and] International Society for Cardiovascular Surgery, North American Chapter.2004; 39: 937-43.

6.   Raju S, Darcey R, Neglen P. Unexpected major role for venous stenting in deep reflux disease. Journal of vascular surgery : official publication, the Society for Vascular Surgery

[and] International Society for Cardiovascular Surgery, North American Chapter.2010; 51: 401-8; discussion 8.

7. Neglen P, Raju S. A comparison between descending phlebography and duplex Doppler investigation in the evaluation of reflux in chronic venous insufficiency: a challenge to phlebography as the "gold standard". Journal of vascular surgery : official publication, the Society for Vascular Surgery [and] International Society for Cardiovascular Surgery, North American Chapter.1992; 16: 687-93.

8. Neglen P, Raju S. A rational approach to detection of significant reflux with duplex Doppler scanning and air plethysmography. Journal of vascular surgery : official publication, the Society for Vascular Surgery [and] International Society for Cardiovascular Surgery, North American Chapter.1993; 17: 590-5.

9. Neglen P, Hollis KC, Olivier J, Raju S. Stenting of the venous outflow in chronic venous disease: long-term stent-related outcome, clinical, and hemodynamic result. Journal of vascular surgery: official publication, the Society for Vascular Surgery [and] International Society for Cardiovascular Surgery, North American Chapter.2007; 46: 979-90.

10. Browse N BK, Mortimer P. Diseases of the lymphatics. JRSM . London: Arnold; 2003.

11. Gloviczki P, Calcagno D, Schirger A, Pairolero PC, Cherry KJ, Hallett JW, et al. Noninvasive evaluation of the swollen extremity: experiences with 190 lymphoscintigraphic examinations. Journal of vascular surgery : official publication, the Society for Vascular Surgery [and] International Society for Cardiovascular Surgery, North American Chapter.1989; 9: 683-9; discussion 90.

12. Raju S, Neglen P. Clinical practice. Chronic venous insufficiency and varicose veins. N Engl J Med.2009; 360: 2319-27.

13. Raju S, Kirk O, Jones T. Endovenous management of venous leg ulcers. J Vasc Surg venous Lymphat Disord.2013; 1: 165-73.

14. Raju S, Oglesbee M, Neglen P. Iliac vein stenting in postmenopausal leg swelling. Journal of vascular surgery : official publication, the Society for Vascular Surgery [and] International Society for Cardiovascular Surgery, North American Chapter.2011; 53: 123-30.

15. Neglen P, Hollis KC, Raju S. Combined saphenous ablation and iliac stent placement for complex severe chronic venous disease. Journal of vascular surgery : official publication, the Society for Vascular Surgery [and] International Society for Cardiovascular Surgery, North American Chapter.2006; 44: 828-33.

16. Kolbel T, Lindh M, Akesson M, Wasselius J, Gottsater A, Ivancev K. Chronic iliac vein occlusion: midterm results of endovascular recanalization. Journal of endovascular therapy : an official journal of the International Society of Endovascular Specialists.2009; 16: 483-91.

17. Raju S, Neglen P. Percutaneous recanalization of total occlusions of the iliac vein. Journal of vascular surgery : official publication, the Society for Vascular Surgery [and] International Society for Cardiovascular Surgery, North American Chapter.2009; 50: 360-8.

18. Labropoulos N, Volteas N, Leon M, Sowade O, Rulo A, Giannoukas AD, et al. The role of

venous outflow obstruction in patients with chronic venous dysfunction. Arch Surg.1997; 132: 46-51.

19.   Neglen P, Thrasher TL, Raju S. Venous outflow obstruction: An underestimated contributor to chronic venous disease. Journal of vascular surgery : official publication, the Society for Vascular Surgery [and] International Society for Cardiovascular Surgery, North American Chapter.2003; 38: 879-85.

20.   Bacon JL, Dinneen AJ, Marsh P, Holdstock JM, Price BA, Whiteley MS. Five-year results of incompetent perforator vein closure using TRans-Luminal Occlusion of Perforator. Phlebology. 2009; 24: 74-8.

21.   Marsh P, Price BA, Holdstock JM, Whiteley MS. One-year outcomes of radiofrequency ablation of incompetent perforator veins using the radiofrequency stylet device. Phlebology. 2010; 25: 79-84.

22.   Hurst DR, Forauer AR, Bloom JR, Greenfield LJ, Wakefield TW, Williams DM. Diagnosis and endovascular treatment of iliocaval compression syndrome. Journal of vascular surgery : official publication, the Society for Vascular Surgery [and] International Society for Cardiovascular Surgery, North American Chapter.2001; 34: 106-13.

23.   Neglen P, Raju S. Intravascular ultrasound scan evaluation of the obstructed vein. Journal of vascular surgery : official publication, the Society for Vascular Surgery [and] International Society for Cardiovascular Surgery, North American Chapter.2002; 35: 694-700.

24.   Neglen P, Berry MA, Raju S. Endovascular surgery in the treatment of chronic primary and post-thrombotic iliac vein obstruction. Eur J Vasc Endovasc Surg. 2000; 20 (6): 560-71.

25.   Neglen P, Raju S. Balloon dilation and stenting of chronic iliac vein obstruction: technical aspects and early clinical outcome. J Endovasc Ther. 2000; 7: 79-91.

26.   Raju S. Best management options for chronic iliac vein stenosis and occlusion. Journal of vascular surgery : official publication, the Society for Vascular Surgery [and] International Society for Cardiovascular Surgery, North American Chapter.2013; 57: 1163-9.

27.   Neglen P, Raju S. In-stent recurrent stenosis in stents placed in the lower extremity venous outflow tract. Journal of vascular surgery : official publication, the Society for Vascular Surgery [and] International Society for Cardiovascular Surgery, North American Chapter.2004; 39: 181-7.

28.   Raju S, Tackett P, Jr., Neglen P. Reinterventions for nonocclusive iliofemoral venous stent malfunctions. Journal of vascular surgery : official publication, the Society for Vascular Surgery [and] International Society for Cardiovascular Surgery, North American Chapter.2009; 49: 511-8.

Chapter 21

The Current State of Deep Vein Valve Reconstruction and the "Trapdoor" Technique

Author(s)
Niranjan Hiremath
Himanshu Verma
Ramesh K Tripathi

Institution
Narayana Institute of Vascular Sciences, Narayana Healthcare, Bangalore, India

Introduction

Venous ulceration in the gaiter area of legs occurs as a consequence of unabated, persistent chronic venous insufficiency. This is due to valvular deficiency of superficial, perforator or deep veins alone or in combination. Most venous ulcers heal rapidly after superficial vein surgery if the deep venous system is not involved, but the results are not good when deep veins are involved[1,2]. Treatment options to correct deep venous insufficiency, therefore, must be investigated.

There is evidence that surgical treatment of the deep vein valvular reflux leading to severe chronic venous insufficiency provides long-term relief of symptoms and heals venous leg ulcers in 65–80% of patients at 5 years following operation[1,3–5]. Risk factors for chronic venous insufficiency (CVI) include female sex, familial predisposition, obesity, smoking, pregnancy, occupation involving long duration standing, tall individuals and deep vein thrombosis. The vast majority of CVI is due to reflux rather than obstructive disease and the vast majority of cases are due to primary (idiopathic) disease rather that secondary (post-thrombotic) disease[6].

However, with the advanced and sensitive diagnostic modalities currently available, this may be changing. Complications of CVI such as venous ulcerations have an estimated prevalence of approximately 0.3%. The advanced state of severe venous insufficiency, including ulceration, is a major cause of loss of time from work that may impact on quality of life and productivity[7].

Active or healed ulcers are seen in about 1% of the adult population[8]. More than 50% of the patients with venous ulcers have a prolonged course sometimes lasting more than a year[9].

Anatomy of deep venous system of lower extremity

Calf veins

The deep veins originate from the dorsal venous rete, coursing through the gastrocnemius and soleus muscles to converge to form the popliteal vein in the popliteal fossa. Posterior tibial veins are formed by the internal and external plantar veins originating in the foot that travel up along with posterior tibial artery along the medial border of tibia. They join the peroneal paired veins to form a short segment of tibio-peroneal trunk vein before continuing to converge with anterior tibial veins to form the popliteal vein. Smaller muscular bunches of veins draining the muscle mass, coalesce to form the gastrocnemius intramuscular venous plexi and soleal plexus of veins. The venous plexus from both the heads of gastrocnemius muscles converge into a gastrocnemius venous trunk that in turn drains into the popliteal vein[10].

Popliteal vein

The paired tibial veins of the leg converge just below the popliteus muscle to form the popliteal vein. It receives branches from soleal and gastrocnemius veins and the small saphenous vein as it dips down into the popliteal fossa. It ascends into the thigh in the adductor canal to form the femoral vein. In a retrospective review, Daniel et al. demonstrated popliteal vein formation at the knee joint and/or proximal to it in 35% and distal to the knee joint in 65% by ascending venography[11]. A single popliteal vein was noted in 56% whereas two or more vessels were seen in 44%. True embryological duplication was noted in 5%. In the lower part of its course, the popliteal vein lies medial to the artery and, as it ascends upwards between the heads of the gastrocnemius muscle it travels superficial to the artery and becomes lateral in its higher course. The popliteal vein contains 2-4 valves[12].

Position, length and anatomical variations of Femoral Vein

Femoral Vein	Right	Left	Overall *
Position			
Medial	57	65	122 (46.1%)
Lateral	61	70	131 (49.4%)
Both	4	8	12 (4.5%)
Length (cm)			
1-5	9	14	23 (9.0%)
6-10	55	49	104 (41.0%)
11-20	48	27	75 (29.0%)
21-30	8	12	20 (8.0%)
>30	2	2	4 (1.6%)
Lowest Point			
Below Patella	3	3	6 (2.3%)
Above Patella	18	23	40 (15.5%)
Adductor Canal	35	45	80 (30.2%)
Above Adductor Canal	66	72	138 (52.0%)

Table 1: Position, length and anatomical variations of Femoral Vein

Femoral vein

The popliteal vein continues in the medial aspect of the knee joint and as the femoral vein just above the medial condyle of the femur as it dives into the adductor canal. The femoral vein courses upwards postero-medial to the artery in the thigh and converges with the deep femoral vein (DFV) 4 cm below the inguinal ligament to form the common femoral vein (CFV). The CFV is accompanied by the femoral nerve and femoral artery in the femoral triangle and which enter the pelvis together to form the iliac veins.

Along the course of the femoral vein in the thigh it receives many perforating veins from the great saphenous vein (GSV), which later joins the CFV below the inguinal ligament[11]. The incidence of single femoral veins is 67%, duplication seen in 31% and complex anatomical variations (triplication or anomalies) seen in 1.5%[11]. There are numerous positional variations of the femoral vein (Table 1). The femoral vein usually contains 2-5 valve stations[12].

The deep femoral vein (DFV) courses in the deep muscular plain accompanying the deep femoral artery, receiving many muscular tributaries. It joins the femoral vein below the inguinal ligament to form the common femoral vein. Deep and lateral circumflex veins join the DFV[11].

Anatomy of vein valves

The most characteristic anatomical feature of veins is the presence of valves. They are present universally with maximum density noted in the extremities and gradually reduce in number towards the larger veins within the venous system. They are not seen in large central veins.

Vein valves are thin, collagenous, strong, bicuspid structures present intraluminal all along the course of the superficial and deep venous system. They help to direct the venous blood flow towards the heart by preventing back flow. This is governed by the structure of the valve and vein wall, peripheral blood pressure, respiratory cycle and muscular contractions.

Anterior tibial veins contain 9-11 valves. Posterior tibial veins about 9-19, peroneal veins 7 and stations in the popliteal vein 2-4 valves[12]. According to Kistner's classification[18], reflux beyond popliteal vein valves is classified as grade IV reflux and holds the key in deep vein valve repair in the treatment of primary deep venous reflux. The femoral vein consists of 2-5 valve stations and reflux in these valves is classified as grade II / III reflux.

Multi-valve repair in global reflux, therefore makes a lot of sense.

Diagnostic evaluation

Clinical Features

Patients with deep venous incompetence usually present with dependent swelling of the legs, pigmentation, eczema, dryness of skin, lipodermatosclerosis and skin breach or ulceration. Some patients may have intractable limb oedema with ulceration. As the symptoms progress the clinical severity may increase to severe venous limb claudication, large ulceration and cellulitis.

A detailed history may reveal previous episodes of deep venous thrombosis with or without treatment with anticoagulants and history of recurrent limb swelling or cellulitis. Thorough systemic examination should be conducted to rule out dermatological conditions that might be contributing to the severity of venous disease. Systemic and peripheral arterial examination should be carried out as that may alter the line of management. CVI is classified according to the CEAP classification (Table 2)[13].

Table 2. Revised CEAP Classification

Classification	Description/definition
C - clinical (subdivided into A - asymptomatic, S - symptomatic)	
0	No venous disease
1	Telangectases
2	Varicose veins
3	Oedema
4 a	Hyperpigmentation
b	Lipodermatosclerosis
5	Healed ulcer
6	Active ulcer
E - etiologic	
Congenital	Present since birth
Primary	Undetermined etiology
Secondary	Associated with post-thrombotic, traumatic
A - anatomical distribution (alone or in combination)	
Superficial	Great and short saphenous veins
Deep	Caval, iliac, gonadal, femoral, profunda, popliteal, tibial and muscular veins
Perforator	Thigh and leg perforating veins
P - pathophysiological	
Reflux	Axial and perforating veins
Obstruction	Acute and chronic
Combination of both	Valvular dysfunction and thrombus

Table 2: Revised CEAP Classification

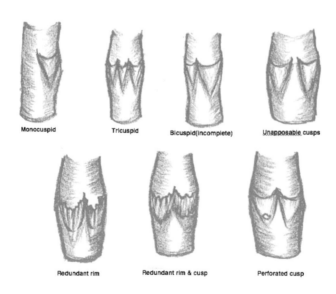

Monocuspid   Tricuspid   Bicuspid(incomplete)   Unapposable cusps

Redundant rim   Redundant rim & cusp   Perforated cusp

Figure 1: Tripathi Classification of Valve Defects in Primary incompetent valves

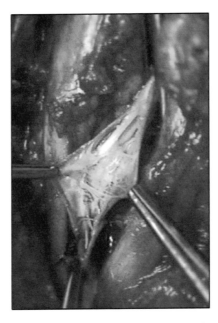

Figure 2: Venous structural changes in chronic DVT showing synechiae and trabaculae

Deep venous reflux is the primary mechanism leading to the signs and symptoms of CVI due to deep venous disease. This can be sub-classified into:

- Primary venous insufficiency (PVI)
- Secondary venous insufficiency (SVI)

PVI comprises of congenital defects of vein valves leading to reflux venous flow, venous hypertension and clinical signs[14]. It can be classified further according to the characteristic pathology of the valves (Figure 1).

SVI may occur following direct vein valve and vein wall damage at the valve station mostly as a consequence of DVT, direct injury, phlebitis or over-distension of vein walls due to hormonal effects or high pressures (Figure 2)[14]. Despite wide spread scepticism, even these valves can be repaired or neo-valve can be created in these veins in a significant majority of patients[36,37].

Non-invasive Investigations

Venous Duplex study

Venous duplex scan determines the extent and the nature of the disease. It consists of B mode ultrasound and colour Doppler. The B-flow mode provides visualization of the flowing stream in real time as it approaches and passes through the valve cusps and has the advantage of showing the effect of flow events on the valve cusps, because both flow and structures are visualised in grey scale (Figure 3b). It can show refluxing valves and this can be quantified including measuring inter-valve distance. Variations in flow velocity and direction are identified below, through and around the valve cusps under conditions of quiet breathing and exercise, with the patient in both the recumbent and standing positions. A reflux time of more than 0.5-1 second is considered abnormal seen during simulated calf compression distally[15]. Vein wall thickening and valve motility and quality can be assessed. Wall thickening appears as bright white walls compared to the normal vein wall[16].

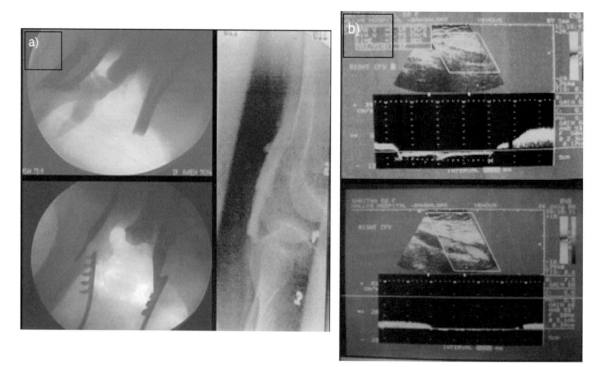

Figure 3: Pre and post Internal Valvuloplasty- a) Descending Venography, b) Deep Venous Duplex Scan

<u>Air Plethysmography</u>

This method of measuring venous hypertension in CVI was devised to measure the three main components contributing to CVI that is venous reflux, proximal venous obstruction and poor calf muscle pump. This device consists of a 35cm long tubular air chamber wrapped around the entire leg. This tubular chamber is filled with air to a pressure of 6mmHg and connected to a transducer. A syringe filled with air is used for calibration. Changes in the volume of venous blood in the leg in different positions that produce corresponding air pressure changes in the chamber are recorded. Hence, the variations in the venous volume in the leg is measured indicating the degree and effects of venous reflux[17].

Invasive Investigations
<u>Descending Venography</u>
Venographic studies may provide adequate conclusive information about the anatomy of the deep

venous system and help in ruling out obstructions as a major contributing factor. Descending venography (Figure 3a) is used to determine the level of valve stations that are incompetent and helps to demonstrate the valve(s) suitable for repair. Assessment of the profunda femoris vein is equally important in determining the site of valve repair or the need for transposition. Venography is not completely specific and reliable by itself. However, when combined with venous duplex (Figure 3b), it can provide the maximum information possible and aid in decision-making. Deep venous reflux by descending venography can be graded according to Kistner's classification (Table 3)[18].

Grade 0	Competence	No reflux below common femoral
Grade I	Minimal Incompetence	Reflux to upper thigh
Grade II	Mild Incompetence	Reflux to just above knee
Grade III	Moderate Incompetence	Reflux to level of knee
Grade IV	Severe Incompetence	Reflux to calf veins

Kistner's Descending Venographic Classification of Deep Venous Reflux

Table 3: Kistner's Descending Venographic Classification of Deep Venous Reflux

Treatment of Deep Venous Reflux

<u>Selection of Patients</u>

Criteria for inclusion in the present study were as follows:

A. Patients with clinical, etiological, anatomical, pathological classification (CEAP) C6 ulceration of leg ≥ 3 cm diameter and present for more than 3 months duration unhealed.

B. Evidence of severe deep venous reflux: Kistner's grade III/IV reflux on descending venogram and valve closure time (VCT) > 3 s (severe reflux) associated with reflux velocities >5 cm/s by standing Duplex scan with patient performing Valsalva manoeuvre.

C. Failure of conservative therapy for more than 3 months, with class II/III compression stockings/four layer bandage + Daflon (Servier International, Paris, France)

D. Previous superficial or perforator vein operation(s) with no current duplex-recorded superficial or perforator vein incompetence.

E. Open surgical demonstration of a repairable, refluxive valve.

<u>External Valvuloplasty</u>

External valvuloplasty is a less invasive technique that may involve either adventitial or trans-commissural plication of the valve cusps. It can be performed by one of 3 techniques:

1. Anterior Commissural Plication described by Nicolaides et al.[19]
2. Bicommissural Plication as described by Raju (Figure 4)[20].
3. Angioscope Guided External Valvuloplasty by Hoshino/Gloviczki (Figure 5)[21].
Raju et al. reported results of repairing 179 valves in 141 limbs with a 3-year competency of 63%

and clinical improvement without recurrence in 70%[20]. We reported a series of standard external valvuloplasty with 19 repairs in 12 limbs with a competence rate of 31.6% and ulcer free rate of 50% at 2 years[22]. Long-term problems like valve station dilatation and plication fibrosis at the commissures, limit the efficacy of this procedure and it has a very limited utility in the authors' practice.

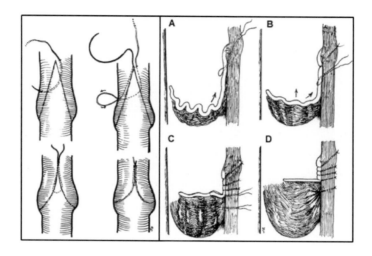

Figure 4: Raju technique of Bicommisural External Valvuloplasty

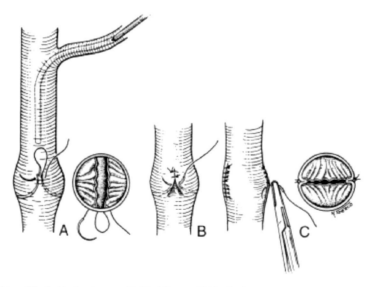

Figure 5: Hoshino-Gloviczki Angioscope Guided External Valvuloplasty

External Banding

This is a method that utilizes an external wrap of polytetrafluoroethelene (PTFE) or silicon to narrow the lumen thus maintaining the approximation and competence of the valves. The external sleeve may be anchored to the adventitia using sutures to prevent migration. Lane et al. proposed an external valvular stent Venocuff II™ (AllVascular, Pty Ltd., Sydney, Australia)[23]. It is made of Dacron-reinforced silicon with an adjustable diameter that is found to be far more superior to Dacron and PTFE in animal models. Many authors have abandoned this procedure because of concern of scarring and fibrosis of the treated vein.

Internal Valvuloplasty

Robert Kistner reported his first description of a direct approach to correcting venous valve incompetency in 1968[24].

His procedure was described as the Trans-commissural Vertical Venotomy (Figure 6)[25,26]. It is an elegant, precise and durable procedure that involved a 'blind' incision to bisect the commissural axis. It requires considerable experience, technical skill and precise surgical judgment to get it accurately "bang in the middle" of the cusps. The floppy, delicate, redundant valve cusps are extremely susceptible to inadvertent injury and hence this technique may be difficult to perform by inexperienced surgeons and in small caliber veins. Venospasm also may occur, narrowing the cusp diameter and giving the appearance of false negative reflux. However, this technique has proven to be very durable. Kistner reported hemodynamic improvement in 60% and ulcer recurrence in only 35% of his patients over a follow-up of 48-252 months[26]. Raju described a supravalvular transverse venotomy technique for valvuloplasty and reported improvement in venous hemodynamics in 63% of patients over 2 to 8 years follow-up[27].

The third approach is a combined vertical and transverse 'T' shaped access to the target vein valve amalgamating the Raju and Kistner approaches. Vikrom Sottiurai[28], who described this technique, reported haemodynamic improvement in 80% of patients at 7 years[29].

More recently, we described the Trapdoor Internal Valvuloplasty in 2001, which is described in detail later in this chapter.

Sottiurai and others believe that the popliteal vein is the gatekeeper of the leg veins and recommend popliteal level repair. Kistner and Raju have recommended repair of the common femoral vein or termination at the superficial femoral level. In our practice, we determine the site of valve reconstruction at valve stations with maximum reflux diagnosed using descending venography. We use two level repairs in patients with Kistner's grade III and IV reflux. We also found that patients who underwent multi-level repairs had superior results to single-level repairs, irrespective of sites of repair. The gatekeeper concept may therefore not hold as much emphasis as in the past.

The benefits of valvular reconstructions are superior in the primary reflux group compared to the secondary (post-thrombotic) reflux group. This is due to intact vein valves in the non-thrombotic or primary reflux patients compared to the fibrosis traumatised and damaged valves seen in post-thrombotic cases.

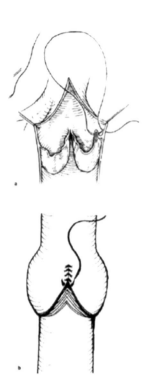

Figure 6: Kistner Technique of Internal Valvuloplasty

Series	Year	Main site	Number of limbs	Months of follow-up (average)	Number competent	Number Symptom Recurrence /unchanged	Haemodynamic improvement
Kistner[25]	1975	FV	15	36-34(60)	5/14	2/15	7/8
Ferris and Kistner[44]	1982	FV	32	12-156(72)	16/22	6/32	10/15
Raju[27]	1983	FV	15	3-40	15/15 4/5	0/15	12/19
Erickson and Almgren[45]	1986	FV	19	84(44)	13/19	5/19	40/42 24/25
Cheatle and Perrin[46]	1994	FV	52	3-54	46/52 23/27	7/51	
Masuda and Kistner[26]	1994	FV	32	48-256(127)	24/31	9/32	
Raju et al[47]	1996	FV	81	12-144	30/71	16/68	
Lurie et al[48]	1997	FV	49	36-108(74)		18/49	
Perrin[49]	1997		75	24-96(58)		6/33	54/74
Perrin et al[5]	1999	FV	33	24-96(51)	22/33	6/33	16/27
Perrin[50]	2000	FV	85	12-96(58)	51/83	10/35	43/68
Tripathi and Ktenidis[30]	2001	FV	25	1-12(6)	35/41	4/25	
Tripathi et al[22]	2004		90	24	115/144	61/90	

Table 4: World-wide results of Internal Valvuloplasty

Valve cusp injuries or defects can be effectively repaired with CV8 PTFE sutures. After the development of the "Trapdoor" Valvuloplasty technique[30], this has become our exclusive technique due to its technical advantages. The trapdoor technique yields an ulcer healing rate of 76% and valve competency of 83% at two years. We also showed objectively that multiple level repairs yielded better outcomes than single-level repairs (p <0.002) for primary reflux, in support of observations made by Raju previously (Table 4)[4].

The Trapdoor Technique

After identifying the incompetent valve station, valves with most severe reflux are chosen for trap door internal valvuloplasty (TIV). In patients with more than one severely refluxing valve (VCT>3 seconds) at different levels – superficial femoral or popliteal – a 2-level repair is carried out. Common femoral, superficial, deep femoral or popliteal veins are exposed through a vertical skin incision.

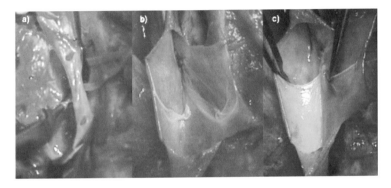

Figure 7: Tripathi Trapdoor Internal Valvuloplasty Technique
a) Venotomy using Trapdoor technique,
b) Incompetent, everted valve cusps
c) Post-Valvuloplasty vein valve structure restored.

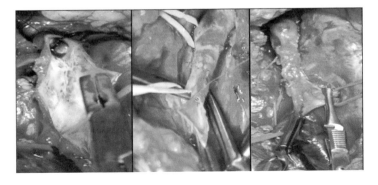

Figure 8: Trapdoor Technique – assessing competence after valvuloplasty
a) and b) Open technique c) closed technique with strip test

To prevent venospasm and vein trauma, excessive handling of the vein is avoided. Where possible, atraumatic vascular ring forceps should be used to handle the vein. After systemic heparinization (heparin 100 i.u/Kg body weight), atraumatic vascular clamps are applied on the vein segment above and below the target valve. Once the commisures are identified, transverse venotomy (50% of circumference) is made from the axis of the centre of one commissure to the other, 1 cm above and below the target valve. A pair of specially designed angled intraluminal valve retractor forceps are passed from the lower venotomy gently to keep the valve cusps away from the commissural axis and a vertical venotomy is made along the more anterior of the two commissures, connecting the anterior ends of the transverse incision using right-angled Pott's scissors, so as to open a "trap-door" from the roof of the vein at the level of the target valve (Figure 7a).

Stay sutures are placed at the ends of the trapdoor and are retracted laterally. The valve cusps now emerge into view, allowing full inspection of their anatomy for any defects in the cusp (Figure 7b). CV8 (PTFE) sutures (W.L. Gore & Associates, Flagstaff, Arizona, USA) are used in an "out-in-out" fashion to imbricate redundant valve cusp edges at the commissure until the cusp brims show no slackness or rugal folds (Figure 7c). The "trapdoor" is now closed with CV7 (PTFE) sutures starting from the centre of the anterior commissure and moving toward the upper and lower incisions. Diltiazem-heparin-saline solution (20 mg Diltiazem + 1000 i.u Heparin in 1 litre of 0.9% Normal Saline) is now instilled from the upper incision and any reflux noted. If necessary, the commissural suture can be replicated and the reflux retested. Once reflux is eliminated, the upper and lower transverse venotomies can be closed, making sure to avoid purse stringing. The distal clamp is released and a strip test is done to confirm the absence of reflux at the target valve in normal respiratory excursions and then by asking the patient to perform a Valsalva manoeuvre in the supine and reversed Trendelenburg (45 degrees) positions (Figure 8 a,b,c).

Results

The world-wide internal valvuloplasty results have been listed in Table 4.

Internal valvuloplasty is a very durable valve repair procedure with 2-year leg ulcer healing rates of 67.7% and valve station competency of 79.8%. The Trapdoor Valvuloplasty technique showed improved ulcer healing rates of 76% and valve station competency of 82.9%. It has also been noted that single-level repairs have a lower ulcer healing rate (54.7%) than multi-level repairs (72.9% P=0.002). One or more valves were competent at two years in 65.5% of limbs whose ulcers healed. Of the valves that underwent single-level repair 59.0% of valves were competent (VCT<0.5 secs.) with ulcer healing in 54.7% limbs. Of the 74 valves that had multi-level repairs, 79.7% of valves were competent (VCT<0.5 secs.) with ulcer healing in 72.9% of limbs (P<0.05).

Single-level v.s. multi-level vein valve repair

Many studies hypothesized that multi-level valve repairs in the same axial system have a better outcome compared to single-level repair[31]. The theory suggests that there will be at least one functional valve station in a repair of two thus improving the over-all outcome. In our two-year study, we demonstrated that patients with primary refluxive disease undergoing single-level valvuloplasty could expect 59.4% valve competence and 54.7% ulcer healing rates compared to multi-level repairs with 79.7% valve competence and 72.9% ulcer healing rates (p=0.05).

Our results suggest that multivalve repair indeed functions better than a single valve station repair in the same axial system in maintaining the overall competency.

Deep vein valve transplant

Vein transplants are used when the native valve cannot be repaired due to destruction caused by a thrombotic event in SVI. Taheri and colleagues described this technique in 1982[32]. A 2-3cm length of an upper extremity competent vein valve segment is excised. The incompetent femoral vein valve station is exposed and the incompetent segment excised. The harvested valve segment is anastomosed proximally first to allow dilatation and lengthening, and is then checked for competence by a strip test performed on table before carrying out the distal anastomosis (Figure 9). Approximately 40% of axillary veins are known to be incompetent at the time of explantation and may require repair. However other options to make the valve station competent must be considered before carrying out this procedure[33,34].

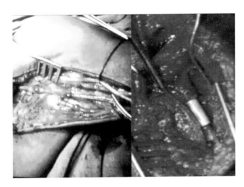

Figure 9: Vein valve transplant and external Acuseal™ (WL Gore and Associates, Flagstaff, Ariz., USA) banding

Neovalve

Recently, Lugli and Maleti described a novel method of valve reformation called the Neovalve[35]. This involves creating a pocket valve by dissecting off the inner wall of the incompetent vein. Early results have been very encouraging in SVI for both one and two valve reconstructions[36].

Post deep venous surgery, patients are given pneumatic compression to augment the venous blood flow and prevent DVT. They are treated with unfractionated or fractionated heparin to maintain a therapeutic range of anticoagulation. Warfarin is started on the first post-operative day with an INR of 2-2.5 for the first 6 weeks, then to 1.7-2 until 4 months after which it is stopped[15]. In patients with pro-thrombotic disease the period of anticoagulation can be varied. Patients are advised to use long term class II compression stockings until ulcers heal.

Complications

Deep vein valve repairs are usually well tolerated with a very low morbidity and mortality (<1%) with many authors reporting no mortality at all[37]. Haematoma and seroma formation may be seen in up to 15% of patients[38]. DVT occurs in less than 10% of patients[16,20]. Wound infections have been seen in about 1%-7% patients[16,20].

Percutaneous techniques

In 1981, Dotter proposed implantation of percutaneous artificial venous valves[40]. In 1990, several percutaneous catheter based valves were developed. Single, double or triple leaflet or cusp valves made out of synthetic or biological materials were developed, some attached to a carrier frame, usually a self-expanding stent. These developments were initially tested in animal models and very few patients which led to good short-term results but very poor long-term results[41]. Some of the percutaneous designs developed are mentioned below:

1. Cook Tulip Valve-Z-stent based venous valves[42]
2. Venpro Valve-Bovine jugular vein valves mounted on expandable stents[43]
3. SIS Valve-Square stent based bio-prosthetic venous valve (Figure 10)[43]
4. Percutaneous autologous venous valve stent (Figure 11)[43]
5. End Supported Stent Valve[44]

The authors studied the reasons for valve stent failures and found tilting, boundary flow stagnation, valve orientation and constraining of valve station as major impediments to successful valve stent implantation[43,44]. Development of vein valve stents is still in its infancy and we await future directions regarding endovascular solutions for deep venous reflux.

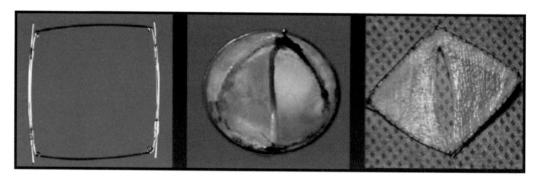

Figure 10: SIS Valve-Square stent based bio-prosthetic venous valve

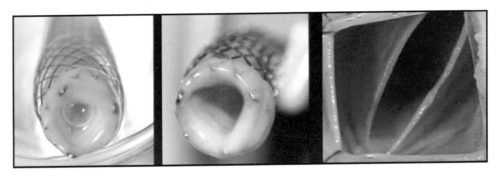

Figure 11: Windy Ipanema - Percutaneous autologous venous valve stent

References

1. Sottiurai VS. Surgical correction of recurrent venous ulcer. J Cardiovasc Surg. 1991; 32:104–9.

2. Burnand KG, O'Donnell TF, Thomas L, Browse NL. The relative importance of incompetent communicating veins in the production of varicose veins and venous ulcers. Surgery. 1977; 82: 9–14.

3. Masuda EM, Kistner RL. Long term results of venous valve reconstruction: A four-to-twenty-one-year follow-up. J Vasc Surg. 1994; 19: 391–403.

4. Raju S, Fredricks R. Valve reconstruction procedures for nonobstructive venous insufficiency: Rationale, techniques and results in 107 procedures with 2–8 year follow-up. J Vasc Surg. 1988; 7: 301–10.

5. Perrin M, Hitbrand B, Bayon JM. Results of valvuloplasty in patients presenting with deep venous insufficiency and recurring ulceration. Ann Vasc Surg. 1999; 13: 524–32.

6. Robert T. Eberhardt, MD; Joseph D. Raffetto, MD. Chronic Venous Insufficiency. Contemporary Reviews in Cardiovascular Medicine. AHA Circulation. 2005; 111: 2398-2409.

7. Kahn SR, Shabklo H, Lamping DL et al Determinants of health related quality of life during the 2 years following Deep Venous Thrombosis. J Thromb Haemost. 2008; 6 (7) : 1105-1112

8. Fowkes FG, Evans CJ, Lee AJ. Prevalence and risk factors for chronic venous insufficiency. Angiology. 2001; 52: S5–S15.

9. Scott TE, LaMorte WW, Gorin DR, Menzoian JO. Risk factors for chronic venous insufficiency: a dual case-control study. J Vasc Surg. 1995; 22: 622–628.

10. Aragao JA, Reis FP, Pitta GB, et al. Anatomical study of the gastrocnemius venous network and proposal for a classification of the veins. Eur J Vasc Endovasc Surg. 2006 Apr; 31(4):439-42.

11. Quinlan DJ, Alikhan R, Gishen P, et al. Variations in lower limb venous anatomy: implications

for US diagnosis of deep vein thrombosis. Radiology. 2003. Aug; 228(2): 443

12. Gottlob R, and May r. Venous Valves. Spinnger-Verlag, New York. 1986. pp.17-21.

13. Labropoulos N. CEAP in clinical practice, Vascular Surgery. 1997; 31:224-225.

14. Burnand KG. The physiology and hemodynamics of chronic venous insufficiency of the lower limb. In Gloviczki P, Yao JS, eds. Handbook of Venous Disorders. 2nd ed. New York, NY: Arnold; 2001: 49–57.

15. Lurie F, Kistner RL, Eklof B, Kessler D. Mechanism of venous valve closure and role of the valve in circulation: a new concept. J Vasc Surg. 2003; 38(5):955-61

16. Mattos MA, Summer D. Gloviczki P, Yao JST, editors. Direct noninvasive tests (duplex scan) for the evaluation of chronic venous obstruction and valvular incompetence. Handbook of venous disorders. London, England:Arnold; 2001:120-131.

17. VanBemmelen PS, Bedford G, Beach K, et al. Quantitative segmental evaluation of venous valvular reflux with duplex ultrasound scanning. J Vasc Surg. 1989; 10:425-431.

18. Kistner RL, Ferris EB, Randhawa G, Kamida C. A method of performing descending venography. J Vasc Surg. 1986;4 (5):464-8.

19. Belcaro G, Nicolaides AN, Ricci A, et al. External femoral vein valvuloplasty with limited anterior plication: a 10-year randomised, follow-up study. Angiology. 1999; 50:531-536.

20. Raju S, Berry MA, Neglen P. Transcommisural valvuloplasty: technique and results. J Vasc Surg. 2000; 32:969-976.

21. Gloviczki P, Merrell SW, Bower TC. Femoral vein valve repair under direct vision without venotomy: a modified technique with use of angioscopy. J Vasc Surg. 1991; 14:645-648.

22. Tripathi R, Sieunarine K, Abbas M, et al. Deep venous valve reconstruction for non healing leg ulcers:techniques and results. Aust N Z J Surg. 2004; 74:34-39.

23. Lane JL, Cuzzilla ML, McMahon DG. Intermediate to long term results of repairing incompetent multiple deep venous valves using external valvular stenting. Aust N Z J Surg. 2003; 73:267-274.

24. Kistner R. Surgical repair of venous valve. Straub clinic proceedings. 1968; 34:41-43.

25. Kistner RL, Ferris EB.Technique of surgical reconstruction of femoral vein valves. In Bergan JJ, Yao JST eds. Operative techniques in Vascular Surgery. New York: Grune and Stratton, 1980:291-95.

26. Masuda EM, Kistner RL. Long-term results of venous valve reconstruction: a four to twenty-one year follow-up. J Vasc Surg. 1994; 19:391-403.

27. Raju S. Venous insufficiency of the lower limb and stasis changing concepts and management. Ann Surg 1983; 197:688-97.

28. Sottiurai VS. Technique in direct venous valvuloplasty. J Vasc Surg. 1988; 8:646-648.

29. Sottiurai VS. Surgical correction of recurrent venous ulcer. J Cardiovasc Surg 1991; 32:104-09.

30. Tripathi R, Ktenidis K. Trapdoor Internal Valvuloplasty- A new technique for primary deep vein valvular incompetence. Eur J Vasc Endovasc Surg. 2001;22:86-89

31.   Raju S, Hardy JD. Technical options in venous valve reconstruction. Am J Surg. 1997; 173:301-307.

32.   Taheri SA, Lazar L, Elias SM, et al. Vein valve transplant. Surgery. 1982; 91:28-33.

33.   Wang S, Hu Z, Li S, et al. Effect of external valvuloplasty of the deep vein in the treatment of chronic venous insufficiency of the lower extremity. J Vasc Surg. 2006; 44:1296-1300.

34.   Ofenloch JC, Changyi C, Hughes JD, Lumsden AB. Endoscopic venous valve transplantation with a valve stent device. Ann Vasc Surg. 1997; 11: 62–67.

35.   Uflacker R. Percutaneously introduced artificial venous valve: experimental use in pigs. The 1993 Annual Meeting of the Western Angiographic & Interventional Society; 1993; Portland, OR: p. 30.

36.   Thorpe PE, Osse FJ, Correa LO. The valve-stent: development of a percutaneous prosthesis for treatment of valvular insufficiency. The 12th Annual Meeting of the American Venous Forum; 2000; Phoenix, AZ: p. 82.

37.   Gomez-Jorge J, Venbrux AC, Magee C. Percutaneous development of a valved bovine jugular vein in the swine venous system: a potential treatment for venous insufficiency. J Vasc Interv Radiol. 2000; 11: 931–936.

38.   Pavcnik D, Uchida B, Timmermans HA, Keller FS, Rösch J. Square stent: a new self-expandable endoluminal device and its applications. Cardiovasc Intervent Radiol. 2001; 24: 207–217.

39.   Dotter, CT. Interventional radiology – review of an emerg- ing field. Semin Roentgenol 1981; 16: 7–12.

40.   Pavcnik D, Machan L, Uchida B, Kaufman J, Keller FS, Rösch J. Percutaneous prosthetic venous valves: current state and possible applications. Tech Vasc Interv Radiol. 2003; 6: 137–142.

41.   Impact of Haemodynamics on Development of Endovascular Vein Valve Stent. Vascular and Endovascular Issues, Techniques and Horizons VEITH Symposium, New York, November 2005.

42.   Ferris EB, Kistner RL. Femoral vein reconstruction in the management of chronic venous insufficiency: a 14-year experience. Arch Surg. 1982; 117:1571-1579.

43.   Impact of Haemodynamics on Development of Endovascular Vein Valve Stent. International Endovascular Symposium, Sydney. December 2005.

44.   Tripathi R, Osse F. Impact of Haemodynamics on Development of Endovascular Vein Valve Stent. J Endovasc Ther. 2006; 13: 34.

Chapter 22

Tailoring antiplatelet and anticoagulants on genetic profile – Pharmacogenomics of vascular drugs

Author

Karthik Kasirajan

Introduction

The Cytochrome P450 enzymes are responsible for drug metabolism and have significant clinical value to optimize therapy with a number of important medications, particularly oral anticoagulants and antiplatelet agents. The cytochrome P450 enzyme system, located in the liver and the gastro-intestinal tract, serves as an important defensive barrier against toxins and other xenobiotics including orally delivered medications[1]. It functions by metabolizing these medications to more water-soluble metabolites that can then be excreted efficiently via the bile or urine. Scientists within the field of cytochrome P450 pharmacogenomics have identified hundreds of genetic variants within these genes in the quarter century since the first demonstration of variants in the CYP2D6 gene in 1988[2]. Since that time a number of clinically important variants in cytochrome P450 genes that alter enzyme activity and drug pharmacokinetics to a clinically significant extent have been identified.

These inherited changes have been associated with changes in the disposition of a large number of drugs. As a result of this large volume of research, individual guidelines that address the evidence supporting the use of specific tests with specific medications for which sufficient evidence exists have been developed in Europe[3], and more recently by the Clinical Pharmacogenomics Implementation Consortium (CPIC)[4], a project of the NIH Pharmacogenetics Research Network in the United States.

CYP2C9 Functional Pharmacogenomics

The CYP2C9 gene is polymorphic with over 11 known variant alleles that result in functional changes in enzyme activity. The frequency of the normal activity allele CYP2C9*1 (wild-type) has been reported to be 78-86% in Caucasians, 86% in Hispanics, >91% in Native Americans, and 97-98% in Asian and African Americans. The most common variant allele, CYP2C9*2 results in a non-synonymous SNP, an arginine to cysteine change that causes reduced, but not eliminated activity, and is present in approximately 13% of Caucasians and 3% of Africans, but has not been detected in the several thousand Asians tested to date. The CYP2C9*3 allele, also includes a nonsynonymous

SNP, an isoleucine to leucine change at amino acid 359, and also results in reduced function. It is present in 7% of Caucasians, 4% of Asians and 2% of Africans. The CYP2C9 *4 - *8 variant alleles have frequencies that are below 1% in most racial and ethnic groups with the exception of *3, which is more prevalent among Asians (~2 - 9%). The rare CYP2C9 *3, *4, *8, *11 and *13 variant alleles have frequencies that are below 1% in most racial and ethnic groups and also result in reduced function, while the CYP2C9*6, *15 and *25 alleles, which are also rare, result in loss of activity. A rare allele designated as CYP2C9*9 does not affect enzyme activity[5,6].

The VKORC1 gene is polymorphic with two well described variant alleles at one SNP site; low sensitivity 1639G, high sensitivity 1639A.

Warfarin and VKORC1 Functional Pharmacogenomics

Warfarin is an anticoagulant that acts by inhibiting the synthesis of vitamin K-dependent coagulation factors. Warfarin is indicated for the prophylaxis and/or treatment of venous thrombosis and its extension, pulmonary embolism, and atrial fibrillation with embolization. It is also used as an adjunct in the prophylaxis of systemic embolism after myocardial infarction. Despite the advent of newer anticoagulants over recent years, the use of warfarin for this large number of indications remains high all over the world, with more than 10 million prescriptions in 2010, just in the United States[7]. In addition, warfarin is a narrow therapeutic range drug whose use is characterized by marked variation in individual dose requirements. The discovery in 1992 that the principal, active enantiomer of warfarin, S-warfarin is primarily metabolized by CYP2C9[8] led to a large number of studies designed to test whether pharmacogenetic variants in CYP2C9 can be used to predict the outcomes of warfarin treatment, and initial warfarin dose. The subsequent demonstration that variants in Vitamin K epoxide reductase complex subunit 1 (VKORC1), the pharmacological target of warfarin, could also influence drug response led to trials which tested the ability of combined CYP2C9 and VKORC1 genotype to predict first dose and predict overall response. For this reason it is important to understand genetic variation in VKORC1 when assessing the clinical utility of pharmacogenetic testing for warfarin. While other genes have more recently been identified which might play a role in warfarin's effects in some subpopulations, none of these to date has sufficient evidence to evaluate for clinical utility.

Clinical Utility of Testing for CYP2C9 and VKORC1 for Warfarin

There is a strong case for identifying better means of predicting warfarin dose. Data from numerous studies indicate that bleeding risk during the first 1 to 3 months of therapy is up to 10-fold higher than subsequent monthly risk[9]. When national data are examined, warfarin represents a leading cause of emergency department visits and hospitalizations for an adverse drug reaction and to significant underuse of the drug in patients for whom it is strongly indicated, in particular, those with atrial fibrillation[9]. For this reason, the FDA has generated a series of label changes for warfarin that highlight pharmacogenetic testing, the most recent of which in 2011, provide specific initial dosing recommendations for specific CYP2C9 and VKORC1 genotypes.

Numerous studies have derived warfarin dosing algorithms that use both genetic and non-genetic factors to predict warfarin dose. Two notable algorithms[10,11] have been shown to perform well in estimating stable warfarin dose across different ethnic populations, and these were created using more than 5,000 subjects. Dosing algorithms using genetics outperform nongenetic clinical algorithms and fixed-dose approaches in dose prediction. A vigorous search for other genetic factors that might significantly influence dose or outcome have not borne fruit to date. When 183 polymorphisms in 29 candidate genes were genotyped in 1496 Swedish patients starting warfarin treatment, and tested for association with response, CYP2C9*2 and *3 explained 12% (P = 6.63 x 10(-34)) of the variation in warfarin dose, while a single VKORC1 SNP explained 30% (P = 9.82 x 10(-100)). No single nucleotide polymorphism (SNP) outside the CYP2C9 gene cluster and VKORC1 regions was significantly associated with dose after correction for multiple testing[12]. As a result it is reasonable to presume that testing for CYP2C9 and VKORC1 variants captures most genetic variation.

The results of the large number of clinical trials aimed at testing the value of pharmacogenetic testing for warfarin, and the number of patients involved in each are summarized in Table 1. Based on more than 30 studies published before 2011, the Clinical Pharmacogenetics Implementation Consortium recommended use of the International Warfarin Pharmacogenetics Consortium or Gage algorithms as the preferred approach for genetic-guided initial warfarin dose selection. Of note, these algorthims are widely and publicly available to researchers and clinicians (e. g. through www.warfarindosing.org). The evidence has expanded since the CPIC guidelines were published, and table 1 includes analysis of 28 more recent studies. Of these, 19 studies involving a total of 8,142 patients have validated the ability of CYP2C9 and VKORC1 genotypes to predict dose, while 11 studies in a total of 4258 patients, notably including 52 children, have been presented that demonstrate positive associations between the combined VKORC1 and CYP2C9 genotype and dynamic outcomes such as risk of bleeding and thrombotic events, warfarin sensitivity and resistance, risk of over-anticoagulation, risk of bleeding and time to therapeutic INR or time within the therapeutic range.

The recent data include two prospective trials which compared genetic approaches to standard dosing algorithms[13,14]. The largest of these, (CoumaGen–II) included a comparative effectiveness research study of genotype-guided dosing in comparison with a parallel standard dosing cohort of patients treated with warfarin in the same hospitals, in the same time frame, and managed by the same clinicians or anticoagulation service teams. An accompanying editorial in Circulation[7] summarized the results of this study as follows: "Nearly all the end points tested showed significant benefits with the pharmacogenetic-guided dosing, including out-of-range INRs, percentage of time in the therapeutic range (PTTR), and serious adverse events. Specifically, the pharmacogenetic cohort had a 10.3% absolute (and 25% relative) reduction in the out-of-range INRs at 1 month, with similar differences at 3 months. This finding was primarily attributable to significantly fewer INR values <1.5, which coincided with a significant 66% lower rate of deep vein thrombosis. The reduced number of out-of-range INRs led to a greater PTTR in the pharmacogenetic cohort, with 69% and 71% PTTR at 1 and 3 months versus 58% and 59% PTTR, respectively, in the parallel control group. Thus, the absolute improvements in PTTR were 10.5% and 12.6% at 1 and 3 months, respectively. This compares favorably with the estimated 5% to 10% absolute improvements in PTTR associated with management of patients in a specialty anticoagulation clinic and exceeds the 5.5% absolute improvement in PTTR for which the National Institutes of Health Clarification of Optimal Anticoagulation through Genetics (COAG) trial is powered." It is thus the case that the scientific evidence supporting the recommendations made in the CPIC guidelines has expanded and strengthened since the these guidelines were presented, and although there remains controversy within the practice community about the practicality of implementing broad pharmacogenomic testing in this context, the scientific data supporting it have only become stronger.

Conclusions

The aggregated data indicate a strong relationship between CYP2C9 and VKORC1 genetic variants and warfarin dose. In addition important relationships between these genetic variants and a number of important clinical outcomes have been validated. These include positive associations with dynamic outcomes such as risk of bleeding and thrombotic events, warfarin sensitivity and resistance, risk of over-anticoagulation, risk of bleeding and time to therapeutic INR or time within the therapeutic range. A number of algorithms designed to predict warfarin dose using existing clinical variables together with CYP2C9 and VKORC1 genetic variants have been shown to be superior to standard care.

Recommendations

Molecular testing for CYP2C9 and VKORC1 variant alleles is recommended for patients beginning warfarin in order to allow selection of the optimum dose and to minimize adverse events, including bleeding and thrombosis. Such testing can also be considered in individual patients who may benefit from the consideration of pharmacogenetic variation as the cause of unexplained variability in response or an unexplained severe adverse event, such as a severe bleed or unexplained clot.

Clinical Utility of Testing of CYP2C19 for Clopidogrel

Clopidogrel bisulfate is an inhibitor of ADP-induced platelet aggregation that acts by direct inhibition of adenosine diphosphate (ADP) binding to its receptor and of the subsequent ADP-mediated activation of the glycoprotein GPIIb/IIIa complex. The drug is indicated for the prevention of recurrent ischemic stroke or myocardial infarction, based on the results of the CAPRIE (Clopidogrel vs. Aspirin in Patients at Risk of Ischemic Events) and CURE (Clopidogrel in Unstable Angina to Prevent Recurrent Ischemic Events) trials. Variability in response to clopidogrel has been well documented[15], and high platelet reactivity during treatment with clopidogrel is associated with important serious adverse cardiovascular events including stent thrombosis[16-17]. Clopidogrel is essentially a prodrug that is converted to an active metabolite in the liver. The majority (85%) of absorbed clopidogrel is inactivated by esterases, with only about 15% of the nominal dose being metabolized to the active metabolite, predominantly by the hepatic cytochrome P450 enzyme CYP2C19. Since this enzyme is highly polymorphic, it follows that the most intensively studied germline genetic variations that might contribute to variable response to clopidogrel are functional variants in the CYP2C19 gene. While variants in other genes might be involved in clopidogrel response variability, contradictory results exist regarding allelic variants of genes encoding enzymatic systems that modulate clopidogrel absorption (ABCB1), alternative metabolic activation (e.g. CYP2C9, CYP2B6 and possibly PON1) and biological activity (P2RY12), and so these will not be discussed in detail here.

A CPIC guideline issued in 2011, based on a review of more than 50 independent studies reviewed the literature to that point documented strong evidence for the association between CYP2C19 genotype and platelet reactivity and with clinical outcomes in patients with coronary disease; specifically those with acute coronary syndrome (ACS) and percutaneous coronary intervention (PCI) initiating antiplatelet therapy, especially those with stent placements. Since that time, three substantive meta-analyses of this literature have been published that have essentially arrived at the same conclusions. Overall, 24 studies have documented a positive association between CYP2C19 reduced or increased activity variant and platelet function (Table 2). Only one such study, involving 112 Iranian patients, failed to find such an association. This literature now constitutes a strong body of evidence for the clinical validity of this association.

In terms of association with clinical outcomes, Table 2 documents a total of 18 studies, of which 14 have demonstrated a positive association with CYP2C19 genotype when tested for either the CYP2C19*2 and *3 alleles, or for CYP2C19*17 in a total of 6,134 patients. Clinical outcomes that were positive for an association with CYP2C19 genotype included non-fatal myocardial infarction, angina recurrence, target lesion revascularization, urgent coronary revascularization, stent thrombosis, periprocedural myocardial infarction, acute myocardial infarction, bleeding events, major adverse coronary events, death and a number of combined end points. In contrast, 4 studies in a total of 1157 (493, 416, 97 and 151) patients failed to show such an association with clinical outcome. The aggregated evidence now includes a significant number of large trials (studies in 1327, 617 and 1034 patients) that have shown a positive association with cardiovascular endpoints in the coronary stent setting. In addition a cost analysis of a subset of patients studied in the large TRITON-TIM trial demonstrated a cost benefit to CYP2C19 genotyping[18].

Negative studies include the CHARISMA genetics study of 4819 stable coronary patients (Table 2), but these are not patients undergoing coronary stenting where the largest influence of CYP2C19 genotype would be expected.

A separate analysis of the evidence that addresses the involvement of CYP2C19*17 is important, since this allele has a relatively small effect on CYP2C19 activity[19], and perhaps in part as a result, a large number of data have been required to clarify its ability to act as a robust biomarker of clopidogrel effect. Several observational studies, post-hoc genetic analyses of randomized clinical trials, and one prospective genetic substudy of a randomized clinical trial has examined whether carriage of the CYP2C19*17 allele similarly effects clinical outcomes in patients treated with clopidogrel (Table 2). The largest trial conducted to test this possibility involved 1034 patients, and showed that the presence of the gain-of-function*17 allele significantly reduced the one-year rate of MI from 11.1% to 7.0% (p=0.045) and trended to reduce the combined rate of MI/death from 13.8% to 10.5%

(p=0.182). In addition, 4 independent studies in a total of 2159 patients demonstrated a positive association between the presence of this variant and the incidence of bleeding (Table 2).

It is thus the case that the scientific evidence supporting the recommendations made in the CPIC guidelines for clopidogrel has expanded and strengthened since these guidelines were presented, and the data presented subsequently have served to strengthen the evidence that supports an association between CYP2C19 genotype and clopidogrel response. Based on the CPIC guidelines, when a decision is made to pursue CYP2C19 testing, it would be advantageous to have the results prior to initiating antiplatelet therapy because most potentially preventable recurrent events occur early; if CYP2C19 genotype is not already known from prior testing, every effort should be made to initiate CYP2C19 testing as early as possible and to emphasize the need for expedited results.

A Comparison of Clopidogrel Resistance between Patients with Coronary Artery Disease and Peripheral Vascular Disease

The boxed warning recommends alternate drug therapy in patients with Clopidogrel resistance (2C19 poor metabolizers) for patients with coronary artery disease in the setting of a percutaneous coronary intervention. This recommendation is based on numerous trials that have studied the outcomes in patients with coronary artery disease (CAD). However, no large studies have evaluated the incidence or outcomes of clopidogrel resistance in patients with peripheral vascular disease (PAD), despite dual antiplatelet therapy having become the standard of care for endovascular peripheral interventions. Hence, the author undertook a study to compare the phenotypic variations in cytochrome P450 2C19 pathway that is responsible for clopidogrel metabolism. A total of 4510 patient samples were available for evaluation. Patients were divided into 3 groups; group I with both CAD and PAD (n=588), group II with only CAD (n=3397), and group III with only PAD (n=525). In addition to the 2C19 phenotypic status, 23 other baseline risk factors were evaluated. 2C19 phenotypes were reported as poor metabolizers (PM), intermediate metabolizers (IM), normal intermediate metabolizers (NIM), normal metabolizers (NM), rapid metabolizers (RM), and ultrarapid metabolizers (URM). Among the 23 different baseline risk factors, Group I was more likely to have heart failure, hypertension, angina, hyperlipidemia, diabetes, and group III was more likely to have renal failure. No significant difference was discovered in clopidogrel resistance (PM) or other phenotypes between the 3 groups (Table 3). In conclusion, despite the black-box warning recommending alternate drug strategy only in patients with CAD and 2C19 PM status, this recommendation may need to be carried over to patients with PAD. Peripheral stent trials recommending dual antiplatelet therapy for PAD patients need to take this into consideration.

CYP2C19 Functional Pharmacogenomics

The CYP2C19 gene is highly polymorphic with over 25 known variant alleles. The wild-type allele (CYP2C19*1) is associated with fully functional CYP2C19-mediated metabolism and its frequency has been reported to be 24% in Oceanians, 50-62% in Asians, 68-75% in African Americans, 81% in Native Americans and 63-87% in Caucasians. The most commonly studied loss-of-function allele is *2, (rs4244285). Other CYP2C19 variant alleles with reduced or absent enzymatic activity have been identified (e.g., *3 -*8). The recently reported world-wide variant allele frequencies of CYP2C19*2 are ~15% in Caucasians and Africans, 29 - 35% in Asians and 61% in Oceanians. The CYP2C19 *4 - *8 variant alleles have frequencies that are below 1% in most racial and ethnic groups with the exception of *3, which is more prevalent among Asians (~2 -9%)[5, 20].

The CYP2C19*17 variant allele (c.-806C>T; rs12248560) is the only currently reported gain-of-function CYP2C19 variant. Its major nucleotide variation is a single nucleotide polymorphism in the CYP2C19 promoter that causes enhanced transcription and increased enzyme activity. CYP2C19*17 is common in many populations, with allele frequencies of ~16 - 21% in Caucasians and Africans, but only 3 - 5% among Asians. Of note, the CYP2C19*17 can be found in rare cases to be linked with the *4 loss-of-function allele, defined as CYP2C19*4B which presumably results in loss of function due to abolished translation of CYP2C19 peptides[5,20].

Conclusions

The aggregated data indicate a strong relationship between CYP2C19 genetic variants and platelet reactivity in patients taking clopidogrel[21]. In addition important relationships between these genetic variants and a number of important clinical outcomes have been validated. These include positive associations with risk of cardiovascular events in the majority of clopidogrel trials of high quality.

Data on the influence of the CYP2C19*17 allele in predicting clinical response to clopidogrel support a robust association between the presence of this genotype and the risk of clopidogrel-related bleeding. CYP2C19 *4 - *8 and *12 variants are rare in population studies, but they all result in "knock out" effects on enzyme activity, and are likely to be important predictors of response to clopidogrel in certain individual patients which otherwise would go unnoticed in clinical practice. Additionally, inclusion of the *4-*8 and *12 alleles would increase the coverage of the Caucasian population from 85% (with only *2 and *3 tested) to ~ 93%.

Recommendations

CYP2C19 molecular testing should be carried out in patients who are prescribed clopidogrel in order to optimize the efficacy of the drug and to minimize adverse bleeding events.

References

1.   Rendic, S., Summary of information on human CYP enzymes: human P450 metabolism data. Drug Metab Rev. 2002; 34(1-2): 83-448.
2.   Gonzalez, F.J., et al., Characterization of the common genetic defect in humans deficient in debrisoquine metabolism. Nature. 1988; 331(6155): 442-6.
3.   Swen, J.J., et al., Pharmacogenetics: from bench to byte--an update of guidelines. Clin Pharmacol Ther. 2011; 89(5): 662-73.
4.   Relling, M.V. and T.E. Klein, CPIC: Clinical Pharmacogenetics Implementation Consortium

of the Pharmacogenomics Research Network. Clin Pharmacol Ther. 2011; 89(3): 464-7.

5. McGraw, J. and D. Waller, Cytochrome P450 variations in different ethnic populations. Expert Opin Drug Metab Toxicol. 2012; 8(3): 371-82.

6. Johnson, J.A., et al., Clinical Pharmacogenetics Implementation Consortium Guidelines for CYP2C9 and VKORC1 genotypes and warfarin dosing. Clin Pharmacol Ther. 2011; 90(4): 625-9.

7. Johnson, J.A., Warfarin pharmacogenetics: a rising tide for its clinical value. Circulation. 2012; 125(16): 1964-6.

8. Rettie, A.E., et al., Hydroxylation of warfarin by human cDNA-expressed cytochrome P-450: a role for P-4502C9 in the etiology of (S)-warfarin-drug interactions. Chem Res Toxicol. 1992; 5(1): 54-9.

9. Garcia, D.A., R.D. Lopes, and E.M. Hylek, New-onset atrial fibrillation and warfarin initiation: high risk periods and implications for new antithrombotic drugs. Thromb Haemost. 2010; 104(6): 1099-105.

10. Gage, B.F., et al., Use of pharmacogenetic and clinical factors to predict the therapeutic dose of warfarin. Clin Pharmacol Ther. 2008. 84(3): 326-31.

11. Klein, T.E., et al., Estimation of the warfarin dose with clinical and pharmacogenetic data. N Engl J Med. 2009; 360(8): 753-64.

12. Lee, H.T., R.J. LaFaro, and G.E. Reed, Pretreatment of human myocardium with adenosine during open heart surgery. J Card Surg. 1995; 10(6): 665-76.

13. Borgman, M.P., et al., Prospective pilot trial of PerMIT versus standard anticoagulation service management of patients initiating oral anticoagulation. Thromb Haemost. 2012. 108(3): 561-9.

14. Anderson, J.L., et al., A randomized and clinical effectiveness trial comparing two pharmacogenetic algorithms and standard care for individualizing warfarin dosing (CoumaGen-II). Circulation. 2012; 125(16): 1997-2005.

15. Angiolillo, D.J., et al., Variability in individual responsiveness to clopidogrel: clinical implications, management, and future perspectives. J Am Coll Cardiol. 2007; 49(14): 1505-16.

16. Geisler, T., et al., Early but not late stent thrombosis is influenced by residual platelet aggregation in patients undergoing coronary interventions. Eur Heart J. 2010; 31(1): 59-66.

17. Sibbing, D., et al., Platelet reactivity after clopidogrel treatment assessed with point-of-care analysis and early drug-eluting stent thrombosis. J Am Coll Cardiol. 2009; 53(10): 849-56.

18. Breet, N.J., et al., Comparison of platelet function tests in predicting clinical outcome in patients undergoing coronary stent implantation. JAMA. 2010; 303(8): 754-62.

19. Reese, E.S., et al., Cost-effectiveness of cytochrome P450 2C19 genotype screening for selection of antiplatelet therapy with clopidogrel or prasugrel. Pharmacotherapy. 2012; 32(4): 323-32.

20. Scott, S.A., et al., Clinical Pharmacogenetics Implementation Consortium guidelines for

cytochrome P450-2C19 (CYP2C19) genotype and clopidogrel therapy. Clin Pharmacol Ther. 2011; 90(2): 328-32.

21.   Kasirajan K. Clopidogrel considerations. Endovascular Today. 2012 July 11(7); 33-35.

Table 1. Evidence for association of the CYP2C9 and VKORC1 polymorphism with warfarin treatment

Reference (PMID)	Evidence/Comments from Cited Literature	Sample Size (n)	Study Conclusion Clinical Outcomes: positive or negative
18305455 19228618 18574025	Dosing algorithms using genetics outperform nongenetic clinical algorithms and fixed-dose approaches in dose prediction.	1,015+292 4,043 1,496	warfarin dosing algorithms
17906972 21272753	Warfarin dose prediction was significantly more accurate (all p < 0.001) with the pharmacogenetic algorithm (52%) than with all other methods: empiric dosing (37%), clinical algorithm (39%).	1,378	Positive predicted doses within 20% of their actual therapeutic doses
21900891	CPIC guidelines: Incorporation of CYP2C9 and VKORC1 genetic information has the potential to shorten the time to attain stable INR, increase the time within the therapeutic INR range, and reduce underdosing or overdosing during the initial treatment period.	literature review of > 30 independent clinical studies	Positive estimating therapeutic warfarin dose to achieve an INR of 2-3, the risk of bleeding and thromboembolic events.
22010099	A pharmacogenomic approach to warfarin dosing has the potential to improve the efficacy and safety of warfarin therapy in children.	120 children	Positive dose requirement among children

22040439	Two Chinese with the rare genotypes of both CYP2C9*3/*3 and VKORC1-1639 A/A were found to require the extremely low dose of warfarin.	2	Positive stable therapeutic doses
22075505	Algorithm incorporating the variances of VKORC1 and CYP2C9 genotypes, as well as the non-genetic factors could predict their stable dose of warfarin with high accuracy	58	Positive risk of over-anticoagulation (bleeding)
22130800	VKORC1 and CYP2C9 genotypes were 2 of the 4 main determinants of warfarin dose requirement, accounting for ~ 20% of variability	118 children	Positive maintenance dose
22161100	Genetic factors are the major determinants of the warfarin maintenance dose	249	Positive maintenance dose
22176621	Validation of warfarin pharmacogenetic algorithms in clinical practice for the prediction of warfarin doses	605	Positive therapeutic dose requirements
22186998	Pharmacogenetic warfarin dose refinements remain significantly influenced by genetic factors after one week of therapy.	2,022	Positive dose refinement on days 6-11 after therapy initiation
22198820	VKORC1 and CYP2C9 SNP variations were highly associated with the warfarin maintenance dose.	845	Positive maintenance dose

22248286	Genetic polymorphisms are associated with variations in warfarin maintenance dose.	297	Positive therapeutic dose requirements
22266406	The study confirmed the association between high-frequency SNPs, VKORC1 c.-1639G>A and CYP2C9 *2/*3 and warfarin sensitivity.	186	Positive warfarin sensitivity and resistance
22321278	Detecting genetic polymorphism of CYP2C9 and VKORC1 could guide clinical use of warfarin to reduce the risk of adverse reactions including bleeding in patients.	798	Positive therapeutic dose requirements, risk of bleeding
22333256	Dosing algorithm incorporating genetic and non-genetic factors may shorten the duration of achieving efficiently a stable dose of warfarin.	126	Positive maintenance dose; mean durations of reaching a stable dose of warfarin
22431865	(1) A blinded, randomized comparison of a modified 1-step (PG-1) with a 3-step algorithm (PG-2) (N=504), and (2) a clinical effectiveness comparison of PG guidance with use of either algorithm with standard dosing in a parallel control group (N=1866). The combined PG cohort was superior to the parallel controls	504 1866	Positive percentage of out-of-range international normalized ratios at 1 and 3 months and percentage of time in therapeutic range

22528326	The study confirmed CYP2C9 *3 variant was related to lower warfarin dose (2.01 ± 0.23 mg/d) requirement compared to wild type (3.21 ± 0.11 mg/d) (P = 0.001). VKORC1-1639 AG genotype was associated with a higher maintenance dose compared to those with the AA genotype (4.06 ± 0.21 mg/d vs. 2.95 ± 0.11 mg/d, P < 0.001).	115	Positive maintenance dose
22571356	The study implies possible benefits of assessing VKORC1 polymorphisms prior to anticoagulation.	557	Positive time to therapeutic INR, stable warfarin dose, the number of INRs > 5, and occurrence of bleeding events
22836303	This prospective study suggests that, compared with routine anticoagulation service management, the incorporation of genotype/phenotype information may help practitioners increase the safety, efficacy, and efficiency of warfarin therapeutic management.	26	Positive time to reach a stabilised INR within the target therapeutic range, time spent within the therapeutic interval over the first 25 days of therapy, frequency of warfarin dose adjustments per INR measurement
22851439	Validation of pharmacogenetic algorithms and warfarin dosing table.	63	Positive therapeutic dose requirements
22855348	For low-dose warfarin treatment, the VKORC1-1639 G > A and CYP2C9 genotype variations affected the pharmacokinetics and pharmacodynamics of warfarin	103	Positive prothrombin time expressed as the international normalized ratio, S-warfarin concentration

22911785	The clinical factors explained 22% of the dose variability, which increased to 60.6% when pharmacogenetic information was included ($p<0.001$);	147	Positive maintenance dose
22927772	Based on CYP2C9 and VKORC1 genotypes, the pharmacogenetic-based warfarin-dosing algorithm may shorten the time elapse from initiation of warfarin therapy until warfarin maintenance dose.	101	Positive mean time elapse from initiation of warfarin therapy until warfarin maintenance dose, maintenance dose
22943693	Validation and comparison of pharmacogenetics-based warfarin dosing algorithms.	130	Positive accuracy in maintenance dose prediction
22990331	Genetic information on CYP2C9 and VKORC1 is important both for the initial dose-finding phase and during maintenance.	206	Positive therapeutic dose requirements
23061746	Genetic variants of CYP2C9, VKORC1 and CYP4F2 are significant predictor variables for the maintenance dose for warfarin, explaining 39.3% of dose variability.	107	Positive maintenance dose
23104259	CYP2C9*3 may be the main genetic factor in hemorrhagic complications.	312	Positive hemorrhage events, time to all hemorrhagic events, risk for hemorrhage
23159229	Modest effects of common gene sequence variants in CYP2C9 and VKORC1 on stability of maintenance phase warfarin therapy.	300	Positive time in therapeutic range of INR

23167228	The greatest accuracy was obtained when the patient's CYP2C9 and VKORC1 genotype was introduced into the formula as the critical factor	185	Positive optimal dosage
23183958	VKORC1 genotype is an important determinant influencing warfarin dosing in children.	50	Positive therapeutic dose requirements
23279643	CYP2C9 and VKORC1 genotypes both have a significant effect on the anticoagulation response during the first month of warfarin initiation in children	51 children	Positive over-anticoagulation (bleeding) during initiation of warfarin therapy in children

Table 2. Evidence for association of the CYP2C19 polymorphism with clopidogrel treatment

Reference (PMID)	Evidence/Comments from Cited Literature	Sample Size (n)	Study Conclusion Clinical Outcomes: positive or negative
21716271	CPIC guidelines: The potential benefits of CYP2C19 testing are that patients with genotypes associated with a higher risk of adverse cardiovascular events can be identified, and an alternative antiplatelet strategy can be instituted.	literature review of > 50 independent clinical studies	Positive clopidogrel pharmacokinetics; clinical response: on-treatment residual platelet activity, risk for major adverse cardiovascular events, risks of stent thrombosis
21786436	Intermediate and poor metabolizing CYP2C19 polymorphism is associated with reduced clopidogrel antiplatelet activity.	166	Positive clopidogrel resistance as expressed in P2Y12 reaction units (PRU) and percent inhibition
21803320	Higher clopidogrel maintenance doses were able to overcome clopidogrel low response in fewer than half of clopidogrel low responders The benefit of this tailored therapy was significantly reduced in CYP2C19*2 carriers. Therefore, these patients might require alternative strategies with new $P2Y_{12}$ blockers	346	Positive clopidogrel response assessed with platelet reactivity index vasoactive-stimulated phosphoprotein

21806387	Patients with two *2 or *3 alleles had a significantly higher risk for cardiovascular death, myocardial infarction or unplanned target vessel revascularization at 1 year compared with non-carriers	189	Positive on-treatment platelet reactivity
21831410	CYP2C19*2 allele carriers had higher platelet reactivity compared to non-carriers.	146	Positive platelet reactivity
22045970	The CYP2C19 loss-of-function (LOF) allele carriage appears to affect clopidogrel pharmacodynamics and cardiovascular events according to the number of the CYP2C19 LOF allele.	266	Positive levels of platelet inhibition and on-treatment platelet aggregation
22075408	A significantly higher on-treatment platelet reactivity was found for patients with loss-of-function (LOF) status (wt/*3, *2/*2, *3/*3) compared to normal-function genotype.	288	Positive on-treatment platelet reactivity

22088240	Urgent coronary revascularization and the combined end points occurred more frequently in CYP2C19 * 2 carriers than in CYP2C19 * 1/* 1 patients (7.3% vs. 1.5% and 8.0% vs. 2.3% respectively, all P < 0.05). Hazard risk of 1 year cumulative survival of CYP2C19 * 2 carriers group was significantly higher than CYP2C19 * 1/ * 1 group (HR = 3.59, 95% CI: 1.02 - 12.87, P < 0.05).	267	Positive angina recurrence, urgent coronary revascularization, acute myocardial infarction, stent thrombosis, death and the combined end points
22088980	Among patients with stable cardiovascular disease, tripling the maintenance dose of clopidogrel to 225 mg daily in CYP2C19*2 heterozygotes achieved levels of platelet reactivity similar to that seen with the standard 75-mg dose in noncarriers; in contrast, for CYP2C19*2 homozygotes, doses as high as 300 mg daily did not affect platelet inhibition.	333	Platelet reactivity Positive CYP2C19*2 heterozygotes Negative CYP2C19*2 homozygotes
22116003	Only the vasodilator-stimulated phosphoprotein phosphorylation measurement detected significant differences in on-clopidogrel platelet reactivity between the wild-type subjects and the CYP2C19*2 (P=.020) and *17 allele carriers (P=.048).	493	Negative occurrence of adverse events at 6-month follow-up

22123356	Carriers of the CYP2C19*17 variant have greater therapeutic responsiveness to clopidogrel than non-carriers, but they have an increased risk of developing bleeding as well.	meta-analysis of 11 studies	Positive incidence of major adverse cardiovascular events , risk of developing bleeding
22228204	Patients with the CYP2C19*1/*17 and *17/*17 diplotype have a lower magnitude of on-treatment platelet reactivity and are at a 2.7-fold increased risk of major bleeding events than patients with the *1/*1 genotype. The diplotypes *2/*17, *1/*2, and *2/*2 are associated with increased on-treatment platelet reactivity	820	Positive on-treatment platelet reactivity, risk of major bleeding events
22260716	Phenotyping of platelet response to clopidogrel was a better predictor of stent thrombosis than genotyping.	416	Negative stent thrombosis, incidence of major bleedings
22265638	CYP2C19 polymorphism along with non-genetic factors were not predictive of clopidogrel resistance in Iranians.	112	Negative platelet aggregation
22285300	CYP 2C19 2* is associated with on-treatment platelet reactivity after 600mg of clopidogrel.	498	Positive on-treatment platelet reactivity

22377481	Event-free survival was higher for non-carriers of *2 allele (94.0% vs. 75.0%, log-rank p=0.010).	95	Positive a combined outcome of cardiovascular death, non-fatal myocardial infarction or re-admission for unstable angina
22390861	CYP2C19*2 allele is associated with an increased risk of MACE in the first 6 months after ACS	1187	Positive major adverse coronary events
22425806	The effect of the CYP 2C19*2 polymorphism on stroke care: the heterozygous form in which interaction of CYP2C19 inhibitors causes further decrease in the genetically impaired enzyme activity is present in every fifth drug-taking patient.	354 patients 221 healthy	Positive allele frequencies in stroke patients
22427735	Carriers of CYP2C19*2 alleles exhibited lower levels of platelet inhibition and higher on-treatment platelet aggregation than noncarriers.	151	Positive platelet inhibition, on-treatment platelet aggregation
22450429	No relationship was seen between CYP2C19 status and ischemic outcomes in stable patients treated with clopidogrel. There was, however, significantly less bleeding with clopidogrel in carriers of the loss-of-function allele, suggesting less anti-platelet response.	4,819	Positive bleeding events Negative ischemic outcomes

22461122	Genotype-guided antiplatelet therapy was dominant, or more effective and less costly, when compared with the selection of clopidogrel or prasugrel for all patients without regard to genotype.	a model based on the TRITON-TIMI 38 trial (n = 13,608)	Positive cost-effectiveness
22462746	The study suggests that genotyping studies to investigate clopidogrel response should include CYP2C19*2 and *3 but not *17 polymorphisms in Chinese, and CYP2C19*2 and *17 polymorphisms but not *3 in Indians.	89	Positive platelet reactivity
22464343	Point-of-care genetic testing after PCI can be done effectively at the bedside and treatment of identified CYP2C19*2 carriers with prasugrel can reduce high on-treatment platelet reactivity.	187	Positive on-treatment platelet reactivity
22591668	carrier status for LOF CYP2C19 is associated with an increased risk of adverse clinical events in patients with coronary artery disease on clopidogrel therapy despite differences in clinical significance according to ethnicity	meta-analysis of 16 studies	Positive adverse clinical events: cardiac death, myocardial infarction, and stent thrombosis
22624833	CYP2C19 genotype is a significant determinant of the pharmacodynamic effects of clopidogrel, both early and late after PCI.	1,028	Positive on-treatment platelet reactivity

22704413	CYP2C19*17 allele is associated with enhanced response to clopidogrel and an increased risk of bleeding in patients with blood stasis syndrome of coronary artery disease treated by clopidogrel	520	Positive platelet aggregation, bleeding events
22785462	The incidence of major adverse cardiac events (MACE) and target lesion revascularization (TLR) was more frequent in CYP2C19 IM and PM than EM	160	Positive incidence of major adverse cardiac events (MACE) and target lesion revascularization (TLR)
22839512	CYP2C19 gene polymorphism does not influence the prognosis for the next six months	97	Negative cardiovascular complications
22929815	In patients on clopidogrel therapy, CYP2C19*2 polymorphism is associated with significantly increased adverse cardiovascular events. CYP2C19*2 polymorphism has very low sensitivity (28-58%), specificity (71-73%), positive predictive value (3-10%) but good negative predictive value (92-99%)	meta-analysis of 14 trials	Positive major adverse cardiovascular events (MACE), cardiovascular (CV) death, stent thrombosis (ST), myocardial infarction (MI), stroke and major bleeding.
22940005	In this unselected, real life population of patients on dual-antiplatelet therapy, CYP2C19*2 was a determinant of thrombotic complications during follow-up	1,327	Positive treatment outcomes: a composite of cardiac death or recurrent myocardial infarction

22955794	Patients with CYP2C19 (*2 or *3) genetic polymorphisms had higher residual platelet activities and were associated with a reduced antiplatelet response to clopidogrel.	149	Positive residual platelet activities
22971905	Among Chinese patients, carriers with 2 CYP2C19 *2 or *3 alleles are more prone to high platelet reactivity which is associated with an increased risk for periprocedural myocardial infarction	233	Positive platelet reactivity, risk for periprocedural myocardial infarction
22990067	CYP2C19*2 and *3 were associated with postclopidogrel platelet aggregation and the presence of high platelet reactivity.	447	Positive platelet aggregation and platelet reactivity
23001453	Carriage of the loss-of-function genetic variants CYP2C19*2 and *3 is significantly associated with attenuated platelet response.	617	Positive maximum platelet aggregation, risk for stent thrombosis
23016454	CYP2C19*2 does not cause significant alterations in the pharmacokinetics of clopidogrel at a clinically relevant therapeutic dose.	20	Negative clopidogrel pharmacokinetics
23137413	A genotype-guided strategy yields similar outcomes to empiric approaches to treatment, but is marginally less costly and more effective.	a Markov model	Positive cost-effectiveness of a CYP2C19*2 genotype-guided strategy of antiplatelet therapy

23148794	CYP2C19*2 status was associated with higher VerifyNow P2Y12 response at angiography (p < 0.0001) and 30 days (p = 0.006) but not adverse cardiovascular and cerebral events	151	Positive anti-platelet response Negative adverse cardiovascular and cerebral events
23150151	The CYP2C19 loss-of-function alleles had a gene dose effect on the pharmacodynamics and composite ischemic events of clopidogrel.	670	Positive cardiovascular death, nonfatal myocardial infarction, target vessel revascularization, and stent thrombosis
23260377	CYP2C19 genotype is associated with response variability and emerged as an independent predictor of high on-treatment platelet reactivity.	1,264	Positive on-treatment platelet reactivity
23337798	The risk of cardiovascular events in coronary artery disease patients with a homozygous CYP2C19*2 mutation was significantly higher than in other patients within the first year after discharge.	506	Positive the incidence of adverse cardiovascular events
23340030	CYP2C19 *2 and *17 distribution had a significant effect on platelet reactivity and identified a group of patients at a greater risk of bleeding.	730	Positive platelet reactivity
23357840	Presence of CYP2C19*2 allele is strongly related to clopidogrel resistance (p < 0.001)	270	Positive platelet aggregation

23364775	The presence of the gain-of-function*17 allele significantly reduced the one-year rate of MI from 11.1% to 7.0% (p=0.045) and trended to reduce the combined rate of MI/death from 13.8% to 10.5% (p=0.182). For CYP2C19*2, cardiovascular event rates were 8.4%, 10.9% and 44.4% for patients with 0, 1 and 2 *2 alleles, respectively (p=0.016).	1,034	Positive cardiovascular events
23429358	Patients carrying at least one CYP2C19 loss-of-function allele (CYP2C19*2, *3) are associated with an increased risk of recurrent CV events.	109	Positive recurrent cardiovascular events, inhibition of platelet aggregation
23431496	CYP2C19*2 allele was associated with a decrease in platelet responsiveness to clopidogrel.	45	Positive platelet reactivity Negative nonresponder status prespecified at P2Y12 reaction units > 230

Table 3. Comparison of clopidogrel resistance between patients with coronary artery disease and peripheral vascular disease.

2C19 status	Group I	Group II	Group III	P-value
	(N=588)	(N=3397)	(N=525)	
PM	16 (2.7%)	81 (2.4%)	17 (3.2%)	0.321
IM	127 (21.6%)	736 (21.7%)	114 (21.7%)	
NIM	54 (9.2%)	221 (6.5%)	39 (7.4%)	
NM	226 (38.4%)	1262 (37.2%)	197 (37.5%)	
RM	138 (23.5%)	949 (27.9%)	139 (26.5%)	
URM	27 (4.6%)	148 (4.4%)	19 (3.6%)	

About the Editors

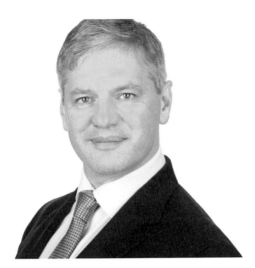

Prof Mark Whiteley trained originally in St. Bartholomew's Hospital in London, and during his surgical training was an honorary lecturer at the University of Bath followed by being a lecturer in Surgery at Oxford University for 3 years. Mark was appointed as a consultant vascular surgeon in 1998, performed the first endovenous operation for varicose veins in the UK in 1999 and set up The Whiteley Clinic in 2001. Mark and his team invented the TRLOP operation in 2001, and have gone on to win multiple international and national prizes for venous research, and have over 100 peer reviewed publications. He dropped arterial surgery in 2005 to perform venous surgery full time and set up The College of Phlebology in 2011 to encourage professionals who treat vein patients to become specialists in the field.

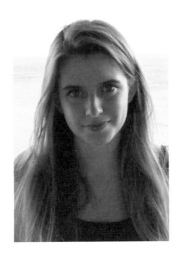

Emma Dabbs joined The Whiteley Clinic as a research fellow in the summer of 2016 after completing a BSc in neuroscience at Kings College London. She has engaged in multiple research projects alongside Professor Mark Whiteley and The Whiteley Clinic research team, and was part of the organising team running the COP College of Phlebology First International Veins Meeting in London in March 2017. Beyond this Emma is a dedicated runner and brain enthusiast, and hopes to pursue a future career in medicine.

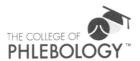

THE COLLEGE OF PHLEBOLOGY™

Join the leading online resource for information on Venous Treatments

For Patients **For Specialists**

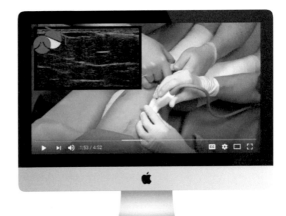

Educate & Learn

Learn, Watch, Understand and Ask about procedures performed LIVE at The College of Phlebology's annual conference held in March each year.

Enjoy Global Expert Speaker Panel, Latest innovations & Live demo's including;

- LIVE Pelvic Vein Embolisation – under local anaesthetic
- LIVE EndoVenous Laser Ablation (EVLA)
- LIVE Radiofrequency Ablation (RFA)
- LIVE Non-thermal Ablation Techniques
- LIVE TransVaginal Duplex Scan for pelvic vein reflux
- LIVE Foam Sclerotherapy
- LIVE Microsclerotherapy
- LIVE TRansLuminal Occlusion of Perforators

Member Benefits

Be found through the specialist search as a practitioner, *plus;*

- Become an MCPhleb – "Member of The College of Phlebology" which you can use whilst you are an active member
- Add your membership and our logo to your CV and website
- Discounts on books & publications
- Discounts on annual conference and courses
- Access experts online and ask questions privately
- Access "members only" learning resources
- *and more...*

Find out about membership options at www.collegeofphlebology.com

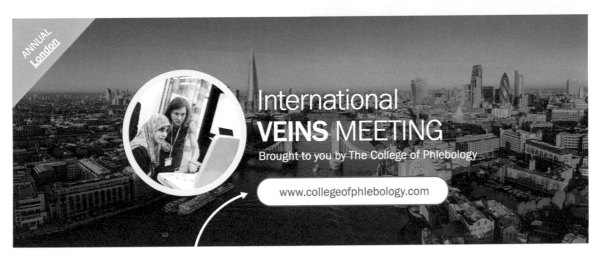

ANNUAL London

International
VEINS MEETING
Brought to you by The College of Phlebology

www.collegeofphlebology.com

Register online now for news of the next conference & courses

If you are reading this you are one of the few among us.

Find Prof. Whiteley, the holder of the keys to the land of research. Take study under him, learn from him and always remember...

Secdum Semfre,

I am the SFP Prince.

Lightning Source UK Ltd.
Milton Keynes UK
UKRC01n0043181217
314658UK00001B/2